TEEN HEALTH
THE NATURAL WAY

by Yaakov Berman

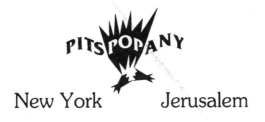

PITSPOPANY

New York   Jerusalem

This book is designed for use by teenagers and their parents. It is not intended to replace a physician's diagnosis and care. The author urges anyone with continuing medical problems or symptoms to consult a qualified physician or other licensed health care professional.

The publisher expressly disclaims responsibility for any adverse effects resulting from use of the information contained herein.

Published by PITSPOPANY PRESS

Cover design: Ruth Kovel
Back cover photo: Sarit Uzieli
Design: Judith Margolis
Illustrations: Betty Maoz
          Lisa Perel

ISBN 0-943706-52-1

Printed in Hungary

This book is dedicated to my mother, Faye Berman.
The Almighty should bless her with good health
and a long prosperous life.

Special thanks to my dear teacher and advisor,
Dr. Moshe Gottlieb, "The" Jerusalem chiropractor.

Table of Contents

Foreword

Chapter 1   Health Hazards .13

Chapter 2   What Are Healthy Foods? 19

Chapter 3   Acne 27

Chapter 4   Constipation .45

Chapter 5   Headaches 59

Chapter 6   Weight Loss .73

Chapter 7   Allergies, Colds & Viruses 93

Chapter 8   PMS 103

Chapter 9   Fatigue 111

Chapter 10   Hair Loss 123

Chapter 11   Brainpower .131

Chapter 12   Recipes 141

Chapter 13   Other Problems
                Other Remedies 159

About the Author 167

Glossary 169

A poor man who is well and has a strong constitution is better off than a rich man who is afflicted in body. Health and a good constitution are better than any amount of gold, and a strong body, than untold riches. There is no greater wealth than health of a body.

— Ancient Jewish Source

Foreword

This book is designed to help you overcome the inevitable, and sometimes embarrassing, health problems you will face during your teenage years.

We all have a general idea about how to be healthy. It usually goes something like, "Eat well, get enough sleep and exercise regularly."

And yes, let's not forget the old standby, "Sit up straight."

Somehow, each of us needs to translate these general instructions for good health into some kind of workable system that will help us apply this sound advice to our everyday lives.

Unfortunately, our interpretation of "Eat well, get enough sleep and exercise regularly," can often cause us more harm than good. As a teenager, here's how I translated this well-worn adage:

"Eat well," meant eating some healthy food...before stuffing my face with choice desserts.

"Enough sleep," meant training myself to get just enough shut-eye to be able to drag myself out of bed, wash, get dressed, and race out the door so I could hop on the bus a second before the doors closed.

"Exercise regularly," translated into jogging to the store to buy donuts and ice-cream.

As for "sit up straight," well, let's just say I considered slouching a strenuous form of exercise which was good for my mother's lungs.

Despite my slightly unorthodox view of things, I managed, like most teenagers, to pass through adolescence in fairly good shape.

That doesn't make me an expert on teenage physiological problems. Working with thousands of adolescents during the past 22 years, however, does. And while teens are as individual as their fingerprints, they do have one thing in common: they all have to get through the health problems that face them in order to grow out of adolescence.

That's what this book is all about. Helping you get through the acne, obesity, allergies, and a dozen other problems that may make your teenage years less than romantic.

So, before we go any further, let me assure you, there is hope. I have treated all the normal — and some slightly bizarre — health problems associated with the teenage years. And I have had a high degree of success.

My basic philosophy is this: The more you understand what is happening to you, the more you will be able to help yourself.

In that sense, this book is unique. First, because it provides you with clear explanations of the various health problems on a physiological level — that means it tells you how the body works, why specific problems arise and how to get rid of them.

Second, I believe in treating the cause of the problem, not merely the symptoms. That's how we get to the source of what's happening to you, instead of just applying "band-aids" to make the symptoms disappear.

For example: if acne is caused by constipation (yes, you read right — over 20 percent of the acne cases I see are at least partially a result of chronic constipation), we must first treat the constipation. Once the constipation is gone, the acne will soon disappear as well.

Of course, I'm aware that if you have acne you want it to be gone NOW. Well, my method will make those pimples disappear, but instead of disappearing for a day or a week — only to spring up somewhere else — those zits will be gone...forever!

Thirdly, the advice presented in this book is based upon principles of nutrition and natural medicine gleaned from ancient sources as well as modern, up-to-date practices that work. A diet based on whole, natural foods is a diet that will build your health and help prevent disease. I have seen this proven time and time again in the thousands of patients I have treated worldwide.

How To Use This Book

Daily nutrition is the most important factor affecting your health. Study the suggestions on general nutrition and try to fit them into your own lifestyle. If, in spite of good nutrition, you experience health problems, such as acne or constipation, follow the advice for that particular problem as outlined in the appropriate chapter.

Treat only one problem at a time. Once you've decided which problem you want to treat, try to determine its cause from the multiple causes presented and follow the suggested treatment for that cause. Continue the treatment for three months before starting work on a different problem.

If you're not clear what's causing your problem, then follow the general advice in the appropriate chapter or choose a treatment from the possibilities presented. Use your own judgement in consultation with your parents.

In general, you should exercise in moderation while using the programs. Don't overdo it. Too much of a good thing can also be harmful.

All the food supplements mentioned in this book are available at health food stores and do not require a prescription from a physician.

A Word Of Caution

This book is not meant to replace professional medical care, diagnosis or treatment. Many problems require medical attention. See your doctor when needed or, if you are in doubt, consult a natural health care practitioner.

The information presented in this book is designed to help prevent, and where possible, treat teenage health problems. Its goal is to help you build your health with natural foods and natural food supplements.

Chapter One
Health Hazards

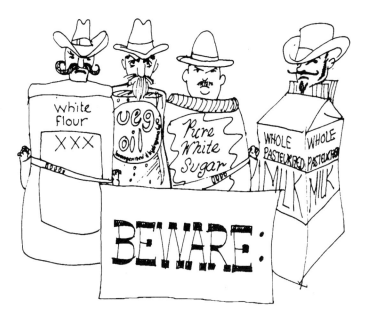

To understand this book, and my philosophy about nutrition, you have to understand that I consider processed foods a form of slow poison for the body.

Chemical stabilizers, preservatives and food colorings — additives that have become an accepted part of our present food supply — are, in my opinion, unfit for human consumption.

The challenge to purify our food and restore our bodies' natural power of rejuvenation is no less important than the challenge to cleanse and restore our environment. Both must be accomplished if we are to be whole again.

The Big Bad Four

There are four basic health destroyers that we should at all times be sensitive to:

1. Refined White Sugar
2. Refined Flour
3. Processed Vegetable Oils
4. Pasteurized Milk Products

Without these four, our quality of life, if not its quantity would be vastly improved.

1. Refined White Sugar

 Eating white sugar tends to lower your blood sugar. Low blood sugar brings on nervousness, fatigue, mood swings, depression, anxiety, cravings for sweets, confusion, and headaches.

In order for your body to burn refined sugar it requires adequate B vitamins and some trace minerals. However, refined white sugar is devoid of these essential elements. The body, in its wisdom, will begin stealing these elements from your bones and muscles in order to get what it needs to burn this sugar.

2. Refined Flour

 In the process of refining flour, the whole wheat grain is crushed at high speed to remove the bran and germ, which are, of course, exactly the parts of the grain that contain the vitamins and minerals necessary for good health. The flour is then bleached and/or preserved.

Breads produced with this flour are often fortified with

synthetic vitamins in an attempt to compensate for those vitamins lost in the refining process.

Eating refined flour causes essentially the same problems as eating refined sugars. Baked goods made from refined flour are just empty calories. There is no nutritional value to these foods. Refined flour also creates the additional problem of excess mucous in the body, which can cause all kinds of irritations and allergic reactions.

The by-products of refined flour — wheat bran and wheat germ — are sold in health food stores. In the last few years a "whole wheat" industry has appeared, making more nutritious whole grain flour readily available. However, be careful when purchasing ready-made whole grain baked goods. All too often they contain lots of added sugars and preservatives.

3. Processed Vegetable Oils

Researchers have discovered a link between saturated fats, cholesterol and heart disease. That's why so many doctors insist you stop eating meat and butter which are high in saturated fats. Instead, they advise you to shift to polyunsaturated fats, like vegetable oils. But don't think that vegetable oils are so healthy, either.

The problem with unsaturated fats is that they spoil quicker than saturated fats. Spoilage destroys the vitamins in the oil. In order to combat the problem of spoilage in vegetable oils food manufacturers add preservatives. They also use the chemical-altering process of hydrogenation which changes the molecular structure of the oil.

One result of this process is that vegetable oils stay solid at room temperature, as in the case of margarine. However, the linoleic acid and vitamin E content (elements that are important in cutting cholesterol) of the oils are diminished and you end up ingesting a chemically-altered substance, somewhat akin to plastic, with little nutritional value.

Cold-pressed vegetable oils, however, are not subjected to heat or hydrogenation. I recommend you use these oils exclusively.

4. Pasteurized Milk Products

Pasteurization is the process in which milk and milk products are heated to a very high temperature in order to kill harmful bacteria. Unfortunately, this heating process also destroys most of the vitamin C and reduces the B-complex vitamins, naturally found in milk, by almost 40 percent.

The greatest danger lies in the body's inability to digest and assimilate the altered milk protein. This protein eventually clogs the small blood and lymph capillaries and irritates the tissues of the body. The body then produces excess mucous as a natural compensation for the tissue irritation.

As a result of pasteurization and the negative effects of this altered milk, many people suffer from constipation, headaches and allergies, including skin problems.

Milk is not only pasteurized, it is also homogenized. This additional process alters the fat molecules making it difficult for our pancreatic enzymes to break down fat.

All this processing has helped perpetuate, perhaps the most common allergy of our day, milk allergy. Over the years I have found that many allergies, and most upper respiratory tract and ear infections can be controlled simply by removing all dairy products from the sufferer's diet.

If you feel you have a milk allergy, try substituting soya milk or goat's milk in place of dairy products.

Perhaps now you can understand why processed foods —

those everyday foods you eat without thinking — may be slowly destroying your body's power of self-healing.

When you read this book, remember that the old adage, "You are what you eat" is more than just words. Think before you put something in your mouth. Remember, no one can stop you from poisoning your body, except you.

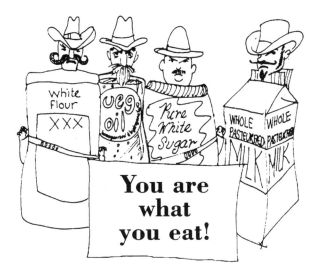

Chapter Two
What Are Healthy Foods?

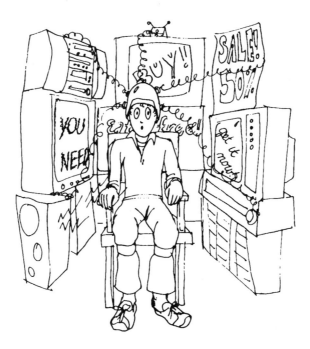

Isn't it strange that by all accounts we are nutritionally starving in the midst of plenty? We have more food and more variety of foods than ever before, yet at the same time more people now are lacking vital nutrients in their diet than ever before.

Of course, everyone *wants* to eat well. Why not? Healthy foods give you more energy, vitality, and life.

So why doesn't everyone eat healthy foods?

Part of the reason is the fact that we are so bombarded with fancy packaging, misleading advertising and artificial additives, that we don't recognize healthy foods any longer.

We've given the food industry free reign to do as they please and have lost control over the quality of our food supply. As a result, our food is grown in mineral-deficient soil, using chemical fertilizers and pesticides to insure sufficient yield per acre. Then it is processed, preserved with chemicals, and flavored with sugar, salt and artificial additives.

To make matters worse, we usually overcook our food, further reducing its nutritional value. We eat quickly, gulping rather than chewing, thus forcing our bodies to work extra hard to break down what we eat.

In the end, we are starved, not for food, but for nutrition.

The Substitution Game

It takes time and a little willpower, but you can learn to eat the correct foods. It's a matter of substituting nutritious foods for empty calories. And it's not too difficult. For best results, consult the table below:

Use this	Instead of
Molasses, honey, brown sugar	Refined white sugar
Whole grain flour/bread	Refined white flour/bread
Whole grain cereals	Processed cereals
Unprocessed, cold-pressed oil	Processed oils
Cold-pressed margarine	Regular margarine
Steamed, boiled, baked foods	Fried foods
Fermented milk products like yogurt, cottage cheese	Regular milk and cheese
Herbal salt, tamari soy sauce	Salt
Garlic, onions, red pepper	Black pepper

Use this	Instead of
Mineral/filtered water	Tap water
Grain and chicory-based coffee substitutes, herb teas	Coffee and regular tea
Apple cider vinegar	White vinegar
Tomato sauce with tamari	Ketchup
Eggless mayonnaise	Regular mayonnaise
Tahina (sesame butter), almond or cashew butter, natural peanut butter	Regular peanut butter
Fresh vegetables	Canned/frozen vegetables
Vegetarian proteins beans, peas	Too much animal protein
Soyaburgers	Hamburgers

The list could go on and on. But I think you get the picture. Get rid of those foods that are nutritionally deficient due to over-processing, and substitute natural unprocessed foods whenever possible.

Proper Food Combinations

Yet, even if you get into the substitution swing you could still be missing the boat if you don't know which foods mix well with each other.

Proper food combinations help the digestion process and greatly facilitate your body's ability to take the nutrients from the food and get them into your bloodstream. On the other hand, improper food combinations weaken or confuse the digestion.

For example, concentrated proteins (meat, fish) require acid digestive enzymes, while concentrated starches (bread, rice) require alkaline digestive enzymes. Eating proteins and starches together (meat and bread) activates both the acid and the alkaline enzymes which neutralize each other and cause gas.

Don't worry if all this seems new to you. As you read this book you will begin to understand some of the processes that go into good nutrition.

Right now, study the food combinations below. They will help you get the most out of your food.

Food Combinations

Do not mix concentrated proteins with concentrated starches.

Concentrated proteins	Concentrated starches
Chicken	Bread
Fish	Grain cereals
Meat	Potatoes
Eggs	Brown rice
Cheese	Noodles

DO NOT MIX

<u>Do mix</u> nuts and seeds with starches.

Seeds

Almonds or almond butter
Raw nuts
Tahina
Sunflower seeds

MIX

Starches

Bread
Grain cereals
Crackers
Oatmeal, wheat
  cereal, noodles
  brown rice

Cooked and raw vegetables are good with almost everything, except fruit.

Fruits are best eaten alone or with nuts, seeds or yogurt.

Lemon juice can be eaten with anything, except bread.

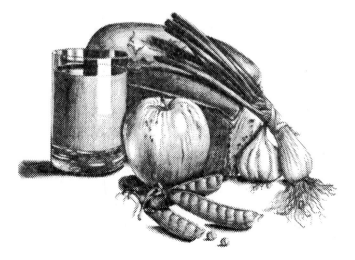

A Balanced 7-Day Menu

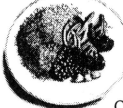

An ideal way to see how good you will feel following a natural eating plan is to follow this seven-day menu plan for one week. Recipes can be found in the recipe section at the end of the book.

Choose one protein meal and one starch meal, each day, for either lunch or supper.

Protein meals
(best not to add bread)

1. Baked white fish with lemon juice & garlic
   Mixed steamed vegetables
   Leafy green salad

2. Soybean tofu cooked with tamari sauce
   Large sprout salad (alfalfa/ mung, azuki)
   Tomato soup with onions

3. Brown rice with azuki beans (rice + beans = complete protein)
   Mixed steamed vegetables
   Three tablespoons cottage cheese

Starch meals
(possible to add bread)

1. Fresh corn with olive oil
   Zucchini & broccoli
   Green salad
   Two slices whole wheat-bread

2. Baked red potatoes with olive oil and hot paprika
   Steamed cabbage and onions
   Large sprout salad

3. Brown rice with steamed vegetables (carrots, onions, zucchini)
   Miso soup as an appetizer

Protein meals

4. Two soft boiled eggs
   Steamed spinach and chard
   Raw salad with vegetable
   salt

5. Lentil soup or casserole
   Raw vegetable salad
   Two slices whole wheat
   bread with peanut butter

6. Baked chicken or turkey
   Steamed zucchini and
   onions
   Raw vegetable salad

7. Tempe and tofu cooked
   with tamari sauce
   Mixed cooked vegetables

Starch meals

4. Yellow corn meal cereal
   with ground-up almonds,
   sesame seeds and raisins
   or molasses

5. Starchy vegetables
   (carrots, pumpkin, sweet
   potatoes, fresh corn)
   Leafy salad and sesame
   oil

6. Spaghetti (whole wheat)
   with soya balls and
   tomato sauce spiced with
   garlic and basil

7. Millet or kasha
   Sprouted mung beans
   Tahina dressing

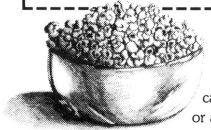

Here are some ideas for nutritious small meals and snacks which can also be used for quick breakfasts or as late-night snacks:

Ready-made soya milk blended in a mixer with one banana and one tablespoon soya protein powder.

Avocado and sprouts or tahina spread sandwich (whole grain bread).

Plain yogurt with fresh apples and cinnamon.

Rice cakes with humus and tamari.

Thick pea soup with crackers (whole wheat or rye).

Bowl of whole wheat cereal with raisins and sunflower seeds.

Instant oatmeal cereal with almonds and raisins.

Corn flakes with soya milk.

Homemade popcorn popped with cold-pressed corn oil.

Cottage cheese on a bed of lettuce and cucumbers.

Soyaburger sandwich with natural ketchup or eggless mayonnaise from the health food store.

Soya ice cream from the health food store.

Whole wheat or whole rye crackers with humous spread.

Raw celery with peanut butter.

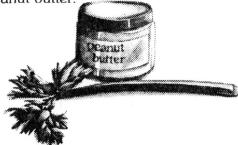

Chapter Three

Acne

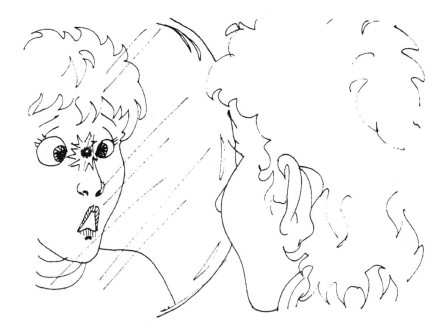

There's nothing like getting all dressed up to look your best and noticing a zit right between your eyes, or on your chin, to bring you crashing down to earth.

Although most teenagers with acne feel singled out, in fact, acne occurs in most of the teen population. In this sense, it's a disease of epidemic proportions, and is one of the most ego-deflating of all the health problems that may affect you.

Rest assured that I have succeeded in healing over 90 percent of the acne cases I have treated by following the simple principles I am about to share with you.

Confessions Of A Zits-o-phrenic

I suffered from an extreme form of acne called cystic acne from age 14-20 — six of the longest years of my life. I thought I would go out of my mind. All I could think of was my acne. I became a zits-o-phrenic, obsessed with the terrible state of my face.

For over four years doctors put me on antibiotics. I had to have cortisone injections directly into my sores. It was painful therapy. Worse still, it didn't work. Then I started getting into natural health, first by reading and then by doing, and within a year my acne and my sores disappeared, permanently.

What Can You Do?

Before I tell you your options, I want you to understand that just because almost everyone has acne, that doesn't make it "natural." It's a disease. Your body is telling you that something is wrong inside of you, and it's asking you...begging you, to listen.

So, you have one of three options:

1. You can try to run away from the problem, by ignoring it. But you can't hide from your face in the mirror. Doing nothing will not make your zits disappear, unless you are one of those fortunate few who have a mild case which goes away by itself.

2. You can try to cover up the acne with creams and salves or use drugs to combat your symptoms. Let's face it, almost everyone tries to cover up their zits. And, again, if you have only a mild case of acne, by the time the stuff you use to cover up the acne begins to have an

adverse effect on you, your acne may be gone.
But in the vast majority of cases, the acne does not go away. And drugs, while powerful in controlling symptoms of acne, can have long term damaging effects on your body.

3. You can deal with the cause of your problem. You can learn what makes acne tick. Then you can follow the basic steps I have outlined below to cure your acne once and for all, using natural remedies that work.

What is Acne?

Healthy skin contains sebaceous glands which produce oil (sebum). The oil lubricates the skin and keeps it young looking. Excess oil is eliminated through little tubes in the skin called hair follicles.

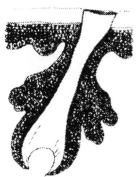

If the sebaceous glands produce too much oil, the hair follicles become backed up with oil. The build up of oil continues until the follicles bulge outward. They become inflamed and before long you begin to see pus-filled pimples, the first stage of acne.

Healthy hair follicle

At this stage it is best to leave your face alone. Don't try to drain your pimples, no matter how tempting. You run the risk of scarring your face. Rather, let nature take its course.

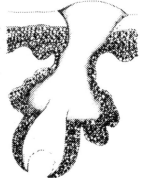

Backed-up hair follicle

Which Came First, Bacteria Or Acne?

Any fluid in the human body that just lies there without being able to get out of the body, soon attracts bacteria. So, when the hair follicles become stopped up and the oil has nowhere to go, bacteria come to clean up the mess. In reality, the bacteria are the good guys. If they would just unclog the hair follicles and leave; everything would be just fine.

Unfortunately, bacteria tend to multiply at a terrific rate. Their uncontrolled reproduction causes irritation and infection of the very area they are cleaning up.

The next step is obvious. Infection means going to a dermatologist for antibiotic treatment. Over a period of time the antibiotics destroy not only the bacteria causing the infection but also the "good" bacteria in your colon. This, in turn, causes *post-antibiotic constipation*, which demands its own therapy.

What all this boils down to is that your bacterial infection is a result of your acne, and not its cause. Antibiotics will not remove the acne, only one of the symptoms. You still need to get to the heart of the matter.

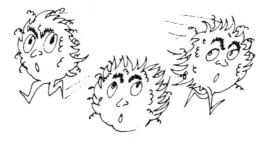

The Real Causes Of Acne Are:

1. Hormonal Imbalances

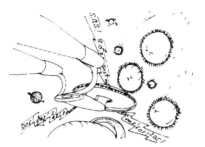

"Battle stations! Battle stations! Androgens attacking!"

His Acne

While the word "androgens" may sound like some sci-fi creatures about to swallow the Enterprise, androgens are actually male hormones.

Androgenic hormones are normal and essential. Too much male hormone, however, results in an increase of sebum oil production by the sebaceous glands. This, as we have learned, causes acne.

The liver works hard to decompose excess androgenic hormones. It's a complicated process, but you can help your liver do its job by adding the following to your diet:

a) A glass of water with the juice of one small ripe, completely yellow, lemon squeezed into it, twice a day. Scrunch up your face if you have to.

b) Vitamin C with bioflavonoids — 500 mg. one tablet twice a day with meals.

c) Vitamin B-complex — one tablet twice a day. Make sure they are from a food-grown or rice source.

d) Zinc Picolinate — one tablet a day with food.

Yet, as every male teen knows, balancing hormones is no simple task. As a matter of fact, you can't consciously stop the overproduction of androgens. You can, however, work on controlling the androgens through the foods you eat.

At All Costs Avoid:

Oily foods   Milk and cheese
Fried foods   Coffee
Margarine   Cola (sorry)
Butter   Too much red meat
Chocolate

But Do Eat:

A large salad every day with lots of romaine lettuce,
raw carrots, alfalfa sprouts and green onions (scallions)
Soya products (soya milk, soya cheese, etc.)

Her Acne

The most common form of female acne is related to the hormones of the monthly menstrual cycle. Many girls experience an acne flareup a week or so before their menstrual bleeding. This is a time of *low estrogen* hormone and *high progesterone* hormone. Usually this acne flare-up subsides at the end of the menstrual bleeding which is characterized by *rising estrogen* and *no progesterone*.

One of the best ways to control the aggravating effect of the hormonal imbalance on acne is to take one 25 mg. vitamin B-6 pill, twice daily, starting one week before your menstrual cycle begins, until the menstrual flow ends.

Teenage girls also produce androgens, the male hormone, but in far smaller amounts than boys. Nevertheless, some teenage girls do have an excess of this hormone and this imbalance can produce acne. If you are diagnosed as having excess male hormone then avoid certain foods and substitute others as mentioned above in "His Acne."

Also, a natural foods diet made up of 50 percent raw food helps to curb the production of excess male hormone.

You Should Also Take The Following:

a) Vitamin C — 500 mg. twice a day with meals.

b) Vitamin B-6 — 25 mg. twice a day with meals.

c) Vitamin B-complex — one tablet a day.

d) Raspberry leaf tea. One tablespoon tea for each cup of boiled water. Drink one cup twice a day.

e) The following foods provide a rich source of the elements copper and magnesium, which are essential for female hormonal balance:
Raw almonds, eat fifteen daily.
Fresh or dried figs, eat 3-4 daily.
Blackstrap molasses, take 1 tablespoon daily.

2. Stress

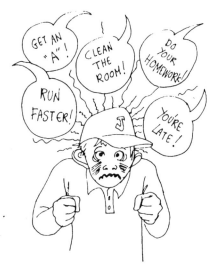

"If I don't pass this exam I'll fail the course!"

School, and the other daily pressures of life, can aggravate your acne condition. Acne often flares up just before exam time.

You can't eliminate going to school — even if you think it would be good for your acne condition. But you can learn to relax. Here are some proven natural remedies to help you.

a) Rescue Remedy is a favorite relaxer that most natural health practitioners recommend to their "hyper" patients. It's made from the extract of various flowers and can be taken several times throughout the day. Just put four drops under your tongue, two to three times a day, and relax. It works.

b) Add a natural rice source or food grown B-complex vitamin daily. One tablet with breakfast and one tablet with lunch.

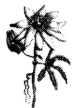

c) Passiflora tea is also effective in relaxing you before an exam, or a date.

Passiflora

d) Years ago, when we still had the entire ozone layer above us, I used to recommend lots of sunshine. Things have changed today. While sunbathing is certainly good for relaxing, and eliminating your zits, it has to be done under very controlled conditions. You have to use some sun block, and limit the hours you are outside.

3. Junkfood

Computer programmers have an expression:

"Garbage in = Garbage out."

In layman's terms, this means that if you program a computer with insufficient data or poor instructions, you will get back worthless results.

In many ways the body is like a computer. It requires food in order to function correctly. Good food. Healthy food. Not garbage. Feed the body garbage and it will throw the garbage out, as quickly as it can. Usually this is through a bowel movement or the urinary tract.

Very often, however, the garbage you feed your body makes it constipated and then your body has only one other normal way to throw the garbage out — through the skin. But, as it rushes to leave, the garbage blocks up your hair follicles and creates fertile ground for...acne!

What is Junkfood?

Most people think that junkfood is candy, potato chips, ice cream, chocolate and cookies. But these are just the tip of the iceberg when it comes to foods that clog up your pores. Most fried foods, margarine and hydrogenated oils also block those hair follicles, as do saturated fats like butter and cheese.

So, what's left to eat? Try some of the recipes at the end of this book or try these snack suggestions.

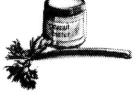

> Plain yogurt with apples
>
> Raw celery with peanut butter
>
> Rice crackers with humous
>
> Soya ice cream
>
> Avocado and sprouts or tahina sandwich with whole grain bread

For Those Who Can't Say "No!"

If you're like most of the teens I see daily, the chances of you saying "No!" to a chocolate bar, or a bag of potato chips, or any of the hundreds of junkfood items available in every candy store, are slim. Even the fear of pimples rarely gets a teen to turn down an ice cream. Of course, substituting some of the healthy items you find throughout this book will help limit your zits. But, ultimately, it's a matter of will-power and will-power, for many, varies from day to day.

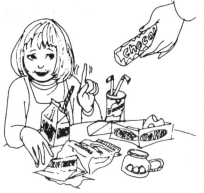

So, for some teens, the only alternative is to try and purify the garbage inside them as efficiently as possible. If the junkfood doesn't have time to do too much damage, then your chances of getting pimples are diminished.

The best way to clean up the garbage is to clear your bloodstream of waste materials. Here are a few tips on how to prevent those sugars and oils from clogging up your bloodstream, and your pores:

a) Take one tablespoon of liquid chlorophyll in a glass of juice or water, twice daily. Chlorophyll is the green "blood" of all green vegetables and acts as a natural antiseptic to purify your intestines. There's an old saying: When you're green inside you're clean inside. Don't worry, neither you nor your blood will turn green, although I have seen many teens turn a different shade of green after they binged on junkfood!

b) Drink one cup of AJT (Anti-Junkfood Tea) three times a day for one month. This tea cleans your blood and, if you put some mint in it, doesn't taste half-bad.

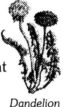
Dandelion

Here's what you do:

First boil 3 cups of water and remove pot from range. Add one tablespoon each of the following herbs: dandelion, cornsilk, and red clover blossom.

Let it soak for 5-10 minutes and drink either before or between meals.

c) Take two garlic-parsley pills twice a day. Today you can get non-smelling garlic which works just as well to detoxify your system (and ward off vampires).

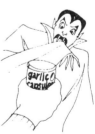

Note: For additional information on the negative effects of junkfood on your system, read the chapter on "Constipation."

4. Allergies

Food allergies can cause or aggravate acne. One of the most common food allergies I find is an allergy to milk and milk products. For many of my patients, years of maternal nudging to "drink milk to get strong bones" has made it difficult for them to kick the habit. Yet, I'm finding more and more teens, as well as adults, who have some sort of reaction to milk.

When I suspect a milk allergy, the first thing I do is to take the person off all milk products for at least three months. Inevitably, within a short time, the person notices his/her skin improving. Sometimes, when the milk allergy is not severe, after three months I allow him/her to eat yogurt or cottage cheese in small quantities.

5. Missing Nutrients

Many teens I meet qualify not only as couch potatoes, but, because of their tendency to nosh while relaxing, as couch potato chips!

Because of poor eating habits and a lazy lifestyle, these teens begin to feel weak and listless. They fail to give their blood the nutrients it needs. The result is a tired, sluggish feeling... And pimples.

After a junkfood binge they look at themselves in the mirror and become depressed, eat more junk, become lazier, and, of course, get more pimples. It becomes a vicious cycle.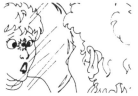

Finally, they go to the doctor, but too often the doctor just tells them to get more rest because, "You may be coming down with something."

Well, the truth is, if you keep weird hours, eat junkfood, and spend too much time hanging around the house doing nothing, you will definitely come down with something, especially zits.

Your body needs certain vitamins every day to keep your skin clean and healthy. Foremost among these nutrients are vitamins A, B-6, C, and the mineral silicon.

Hoẁ To Get The Nutrients You Need

There are some important sources of nutrients which I have found help keep your skin healthy. Try them, diligently, and you will get results:

a) Eat fresh or frozen fish at least three times a week. Natural oils contained in the fish reduce fats in the blood. Bake the fish with tomato sauce, lemon or onions. Fish oils are high in Vitamin A.

b) High fiber foods like dried prunes, romaine lettuce, carrots and wheat or oat bran eaten daily will help flush out your bowels. Remember, when garbage has a clear path out of your system, it won't try to force its way out via your skin.

c) Oatmeal cereal (the kind sold in health food stores) is a rich source of the mineral silicon which is essential for healthy, vibrant skin. Eat a heaping bowl at least three times a week.

After I had suffered from severe acne for four years, a natural health practitioner in Arizona told me to go to an abandoned field and cut down bushels of oat straw. He showed me how to make the straw into a tea. I actually bathed in oat straw tea and got the first relief ever from my condition. Of course, going to Arizona, if you don't live there already, may be inconvenient (most school lunch breaks are no more than one hour). So, instead, I strongly advise eating oatmeal cereal. It is great for the skin.

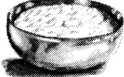

d) Drink raw carrot juice. It is a rich source of beta-carotene which is the substance the body uses to make vitamin A. What apples do for doctors (keep them away), carrots do for dermatologists!

e) Take the following pills daily:

1. Vitamin A — 10,000 IU once daily with meals.
2. Vitamin C — 500 mg. one tablet twice a day with meals. Make sure the vitamin C lists bioflavonoids as one of the ingredients.

6. Shower Shyness

I am amazed at how many teens (mostly boys) think that water is only for drinking or for sprinkling the lawn. My first piece of advice to them is — shower daily!

Daily showers get rid of the sweat and dirt that build up on your skin every day. But, the truth is that even daily showers have to be taken at the proper time.

If you have just finished a gym class and you are too rushed to shower, you are setting the stage for acne. Sweat and oils that remain on the skin will block the hair follicles. Showering hours later may be too late to undo the damage to your skin.

When you shower use a hard sponge or bath brush and rub your skin, vigorously. If you like a hot shower, that's okay, but always finish with cool water. Hot water, over an extended time, causes inactivity and laziness of the skin.

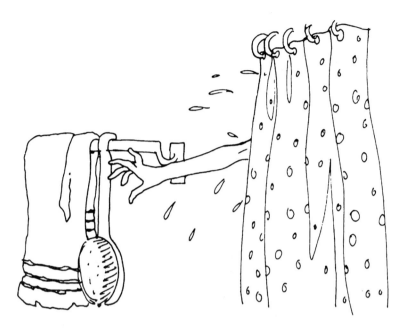

Ocean Water Zaps The Zits

Most people notice a dramatic improvement in their acne condition when they go to the beach. The ocean salts draw out poisons from the skin's pores. These waters are nature's "elixir of life" and, together with the sun's rays, rejuvenate the skin.

Of course, the hole in the ozone layer has forced us to be very careful when going into the sun during the afternoon hours. But, the ocean waters, even in the evening, are just as helpful in combating acne as they are during the heat of the day.

Remember, however, that while heat and the salt water are good for clearing your acne, dampness will destroy any benefits the heat and water may bring you. Don't forget to dry yourself well and stay out of damp bungalows and summer homes. They could be harmful to your skin's health, especially if you are allergic to molds and mildew.

7. Improper Skin Care

The first thing most teens do when they see a pimple is head for the medicine chest. It's cover-up time! The rule of thumb seems to be that if you don't see it, it isn't there.

But of course, it is there. And growing.

If you use synthetic lotions and chemicals you are not just covering up the pimples, you are choking your skin. That's because your skin is alive and needs to breathe. The chemicals you smear on are absorbed through the skin and carried into your blood stream. Many of them have ingredients that aggravate your already toxic condition. Over time, some of these lotions even add to the back up in your hair follicles and cause more trouble.

Ultimately, all you accomplish with all these creams and lotions is to give acne a stronger anchor into your ailing skin.

Help For Your Skin

That's not to say that you have to look pimply while you battle acne. There are natural gels and oils that can help you reduce the outward signs of your acne condition:

During the day, use aloe vera gel. It rejuvenates the skin without clogging the hair follicles. At night, try Vitamin E oil to heal broken skin. Both these ingredients go a long way in softening up already scarred areas and preventing new scar tissue from accumulating on your face.

Of course, there are those determined to absolutely, positively hide their acne, and they don't care about the long term effects. If you are one of these people then I have some advice on how to protect your skin from the cover-up cream barrage.

Before putting on any cream or lotion dab one of the following antiseptic washes to the affected area:

a) Apple cider vinegar — one teaspoon in a glass of water.

b) Herbal thyme tea — one tablespoon in a glass of boiled water (let it cool down before applying).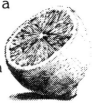

c) Lemon water — juice of one lemon in a glass of water.

Chapter Four

Constipation

I tell all my patients that it is important to have a bowel movement every day. Being "regular" is an indication that your digestive system is operating correctly. Being constipated is an indication that something is wrong.

Unfortunately, almost everyone, at some time in their life, becomes constipated. There are lots of over-the-counter fast-acting laxatives you can take to get rid of the garbage that may stop-up your intestines. I call them "Rotor Rooter" medicines because like the plumbing company of the same name, they unclog your drain swiftly and efficiently.

But they don't get to the root of your problem. As a matter of fact, by making you "feel" good, they may mask some rather serious problems.

To understand the causes of constipation you need to understand a little about what happens to your food when it goes through your large intestine. (Don't panic! It's just two paragraphs.)

The Wave

The bowel, or large intestine, is composed of several layers of muscle that move waste material out of your body. If you've ever watched a football game, you've seen the people in the stands perform what is called "the wave." First one group of people raise their hands, stand up and sit down just as a second group of people next to them do the same thing. The impression you get is that of a wave gently rolling through the stands.

That's how the large intestines move the waste material out of your body. It's a wave-like motion called the peristaltic wave. The muscles of the colon are controlled by two different types of nerves which regulate this movement. The parasympathetic nerves keep the muscles moving and the sympathetic nerves slow the muscles down.

Here are the nine most common reasons you may be constipated:

1. Stress Overload

When you are faced with any extreme physical or emotional stress, for example, a barrage of exams one after the other, your body concentrates all its energy into coping with the emergency.

In the process the sympathetic nervous system, which slows down the muscles in your colon, begins to shut down your entire digestive system. If you have to stay up late night after night to study, your brain, heart, and other muscles are activated, while your body puts all its digestive functions on hold.

When your sympathetic nervous system operates at this high speed too much of the time, it literally overpowers your parasympathetic nervous system. The peristaltic wave stops. Waste material sits in your colon. And you become constipated.

Getting "Regular"

You must reduce stress levels as soon as possible in order to re-awaken the parasympathetic system. Some people practice yoga or Tai-Chi to induce relaxation. Others take a bath or deep breaths or simply focus. The important thing is to relax your body and stop its headlong rush. You have to "hang loose" for awhile.

The following foods and health supplements will also help you along the path to regularity:

a) Magnesium oxide — 250 mg. one pill daily at breakfast. It relaxes the sympathetic nerves. Magnesium has been nicknamed the "laxative" mineral.

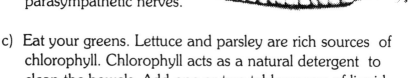

b) Eat more fresh fruits and vegetables. They help activate your parasympathetic nerves.

c) Eat your greens. Lettuce and parsley are rich sources of chlorophyll. Chlorophyll acts as a natural detergent to clean the bowels. Add one or two tablespoons of liquid chlorophyll to water, juice, or tea each day.

2. Lack of Exercise

If you don't exercise, and continue to eat unbalanced meals, after a while the large intestine loses its muscle tone and the peristaltic wave becomes irregular and lazy.

Therefore, if you have the time, take up a sport. If you feel you lack the coordination to get into sports, or are just shy about getting onto the courts, try one or more of these exercises:

a) Lay flat on the floor and make bicycle movements with your legs for five minutes.

Then grab both knees and bring them to your chest. Hold this position for two minutes and relax.

b) Practice the "cat stretch," called "the cobra" in yoga:

1. Bend over, so that the palms of your hand are touching the floor well in front of you, shoulder width apart. The soles of your feet should be flat on the floor. Bend your knees if you need to.

2. Get your tush as high up in the air as you can. Now, swing your chest down and forward. Keep your head up. Swing your tush down and then up.

3. You'll feel the pull in your lower back. Ten of these daily is sufficient to awaken the parasympathetic nerve centers in the lower back.

3. Lack Of Bile

The role of bile, which is produced by the liver, and released by the gallbladder, is to break down fats and aid in their absorption into the bloodstream. It also lubricates the bowel wall, helping the peristaltic wave to function more efficiently.

If your liver doesn't produce the required bile, or your gallbladder does not release its stored bile, fats do not get absorbed into your bloodstream. The bowel wall does not get properly lubricated. And you become constipated.

How To Get Bile into Your System

a) Carrots and carrot juice relax the gallbladder ducts, inducing them to release stored-up bile. Drink one glass of carrot juice — 75% juice and 25% water — a day.

b) Add one or two tablespoons of unprocessed cold-pressed olive oil to your salad each day. It stimulates the liver to produce more bile.

c) Red beets and their green leaves are a strong stimulant. Shred the raw beets and add them to salad. Cook the greens and add them to soup.

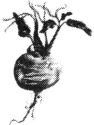

Red beet with leaves

4. Poor Bowel Flora

The bowel contains both healthy and potentially harmful bacteria. The healthy bacteria help decompose foods that cannot be digested by the body, like wheat bran.

The harmful bacteria produce smelly gases. And if that's not bad enough, they can also cause allergic reactions due to histamine production. (See the chapter on Allergies.)

Grow Healthy Bacteria

There are several proven ways to increase the number of healthy bacteria in your colon:

a) Eat sour pickles and non-vinegar based sauerkraut.

b) Add Miso, a product combination of soy, salt, wheat and water, to any soup, stew or casserole.

c) Eat high fiber foods and wheat bran. They help cleanse

the large intestine of harmful bacteria. One tablespoon of wheat bran on your breakfast cereal is an ideal way to start the morning.

d) Acidophilus are healthy bacteria. Take one acidophilus capsule in the morning and another at bedtime. This will help replenish the good bacteria in your digestive tract.

5. Lack Of Fiber

Fiber is the indigestible portion of the foods you eat. It gives your stool bulk and sweeps the colon clean as it passes through. If you lack fiber, your bowel will not function efficiently and you will become constipated.

Recent studies show a tentative link between a lack of fiber and the onset of colon cancer. The National Cancer Institute recommends a high-fiber diet.

However, you should add extra fiber to your diet slowly, over a period of about four weeks, to give your system a chance to adapt. Caution: Some people experience gas during the first few weeks of adding fiber to their diet.

Bulk Up For Safety

There are a number of ways for you to get the fiber you need:

a) Eat more whole grain cereals and raw vegetables, especially leafy vegetables.

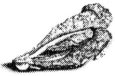

b) Add wheat bran to your breakfast cereal.

c) Take alfalfa pills. One or two pills with each meal help to sweep the bowels clean. If you become gaseous from the pills cut down the dosage.

6. Gassy Foods

Beans are just one type of food that produces excess gas. A number of foods contain carbohydrates which the body cannot easily decompose, causing gas. The "three Cs": cabbage, cauliflower, and corn, among many others, are gas-producing.

Neutralizing Gas

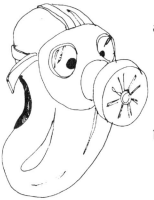

a) Don't eat more than four or five tablespoons of beans at a meal. Before you cook them soak them overnight. This helps to de-gas them.

b) Take one teaspoon of apple cider vinegar in a glass of water before a meal. It helps by breaking up gas pockets in the bowel.

7. Too Little Water

I've mentioned how bile helps lubricate the bowel. But the bowel also needs a certain amount of liquid to keep the peristaltic wave moving at an even keel. Here's what you can do to make sure your bowel runs smoothly:

a) Drink one cup of water for each 16 pounds of body weight. If, for example, you weigh 160 pounds you should drink 10 glasses of water per day.

b) Check your urine. If you are drinking enough liquids,

your urine should be odorless and clear or very light in color.

c) Don't drink with meals. It dilutes the natural digestive juices of the stomach and it also pushes the food through the stomach too fast. Drink either before meals or wait two hours after meals.

8. Failure To Set Your Body Clock

There is an internal body clock that sets the rhythm for many things in your life. Your body "knows" when it's time to eat, and when it's time to sleep. More than likely, you experience daily highs and lows at the same time each day.

There is an internal clock for bowel movements as well. And if you are tuned into your body, you will note that you "do your thing" at about the same time each day.

However, stress and severe pressures from school or work can change your body clock. Your internal rhythm can be out of sync if you are forced to switch your daily schedule too often. This may lead to constipation.

How To Set Your Body Clock

You cannot set or re-set your internal clock by simply wishing it. We are creatures of habit. So it is habit that sets our internal rhythms.

Therefore, to get your biological clock into a routine do the following:

a) Go to sleep at exactly the same time every night for six nights in a row and get up (by alarm clock or parental nudging) at the same time each morning.

b) Try to go to the bathroom at the same time each day. In a short time you will find your bowel rhythms will be back in working order.

9. Poor Food Combinations

Even the most nutritious natural foods can cause gas and constipation if you ignore the rules of proper food combining. The basic rules are outlined below.

What you should remember is that certain foods, such as starches, need an alkaline environment in order to be broken down and used efficiently by the body. Other foods, such as proteins, require an acid environment before the body can get the most out of them.

When you eat bread and meat together the alkaline and acid enzymes cancel each other out, making digestion much more difficult, and constipation more likely. That's why I recommend that you separate proteins (meat, fish, eggs, etc.) and starches (bread, rice, potatoes, etc.), eating each at separate meals.

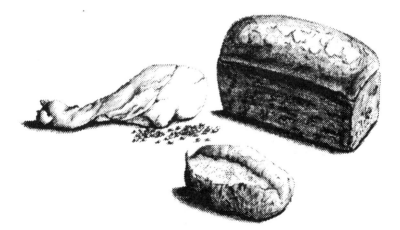

Summary Chart: Constipation

Cause	Treatment
Stress Overload	Magnesium Oxide 250 mg. Eat fresh fruits and vegetables Chlorophyll one-two tablespoons daily
Lack of Bile	Carrot juice daily One-two tablespoons olive oil daily Raw beets/cooked beet greens
Lack of Exercise	Exercise
Poor Bowel Flora	Pickles/non-vinegar sauerkraut Miso One tablespoon wheat bran in cereal Acidophilus capsules
Lack of Fiber	Whole grain cereal Vegetables Wheat bran Alfalfa pills

Summary Chart: Constipation (con't)

Cause	Treatment
Gassy Foods	Limit beans to four-five tablespoons daily Apple cider vinegar before meals
Too Little Water	Drink one cup liquid per each 16 pounds Don't drink with meals
Body Clock	Reset your internal clock
Poor Food Combinations	Eat starches and proteins at separate meals

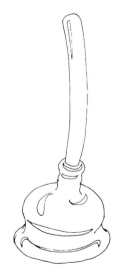

A Food Plan To Fight Constipation

Today, people pop laxatives almost as often as they take pain killers. Ideally, you should break the laxative habit. Whether natural or over-the-counter, laxatives can eventually irritate or damage the bowel, or push it to work too hard.

The food plan below helps you fight constipation. It will also let you kick the laxative habit, giving you one less thing to worry about.

Early Morning Cocktail (choose one)

a) One teaspoon of dried rosemary steeped in a cup of boiled water.

b) Squeeze one small, completely yellow lemon into a cup of water and sweeten with one teaspoon of honey.

c) One large glass of prune juice. (That should do it!)

Breakfast (choose one)

a) The Mt. Vesuvius: soak two prunes, two figs, one teaspoon of raisins, and a tablespoon of wheat bran, overnight. Add enough water to submerge the fruits. In the morning eat the mixture and drink the water.

Watch out for the explosion!

b) Try a bowl of yellow cornmeal cereal with tahina, sweetened with molasses.

c) Whole wheat cereal with dried fruits or molasses.

d) Whole wheat toast with tahina or almond butter and fresh salad.

e) Yogurt (preferably from goat's milk) with fresh fruit or granola. Soya milk with granola is good too!

Lunch (choose one)

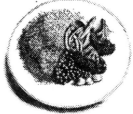

a) Cooked vegetables with fresh raw vegetables, seasoned with tamari sauce.

b) Cooked vegetables, seasoned with tamari sauce, and cereal made of millet, bulgur wheat or kasha.

Supper (choose one)

a) Fresh fish with sprout salad and cooked vegetables.

b) Fresh fish with fermented vegetables (non-vinegar pickles or non-vinegar sauerkraut).

c) Baked potatoes with one tablespoon olive oil and vegetable soup and salad.

You can switch supper with lunch if you like. Try snacking on carrot or celery sticks or fresh fruit during the day.

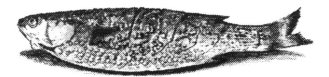

Anti-Constipation Laxatives

The following are useful as gentle laxatives and can be used as supplements to your regular daily diet. They are not addictive and can be taken as needed. Best of all, they will not damage your bowel.

a) Fruit juices, especially grape and pear juices.

b) Prunes, figs, and raisins.

c) Molasses.

d) Wheat bran or alfalfa tablets — up to two pills per meal.

e) Acidophilus capsules — one early morning and one before bed.

f) Magnesium chelate — one pill per day at breakfast.

If all else fails, Mother Nature has a secret weapon. It's an herbal bark called, Cascara Sagrada, and it means "sacred bark." Take one capsule at night before bed with a glass of water.

Chapter Five

Headaches

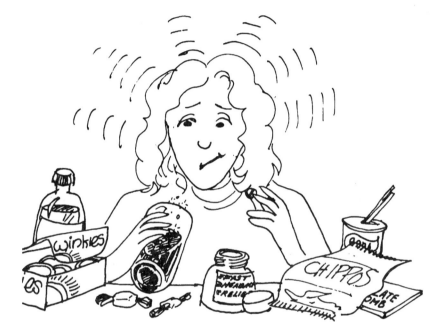

When Tanya came to me she was rubbing the sides of her head.

"I'll be all right in a moment," she assured me as she popped two pain killers into her mouth. Sure enough, within moments, she seemed more relaxed. The pained expression around her eyes was gone.

"Do you mind if I nosh on something?" she asked, opening a package of cookies she had taken out of her purse. "I came straight from school, and I'm starved. You wouldn't have any cola around here, would you? These things always make me thirsty."

Tanya then asked me to explain the cause of her nagging headaches.

"How many pain killers do you take a day?" I inquired.

"I only take them when I feel a headache coming on. Sometimes I take six or eight a day, sometimes only two. It depends."

"Well, it seems to me, Tanya," I told her, "that you don't have a headache problem, you're suffering from a pain killer deficiency!"

In a way this was true. Pain killers suppress the pain of a headache, but they don't treat the cause. They make you feel good. But, if you don't investigate and eliminate the root of your headache problem, you may end up being a pain killer junkie like Tanya.

Of course, it was easy to see that Tanya was bringing on her headaches with her 1-2 combination of cake and cola. It took a while, but eventually Tanya was able to understand that her sugar levels were at the root of her problem. And, of course, her headaches stopped.

Types Of Headaches

Most headaches fall into one of two categories: acute and chronic.

Acute Headaches

Acute headaches are one-shot deals. They happen rarely and, while they may be very painful, it is almost impossible to diagnose their origin.

Everyone gets an acute headache at sometime in their lives. The headache can last for a few moments or for a long time. In any case, if you get an acute headache, try one or both of these herbal remedies. They have worked wonders with many of my patients.

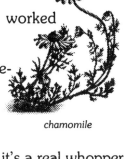
chamomile

a) Acute Killer Tea Mix — add one table-spoon each of chamomile, vervain, passion flower and lemon balm to three cups of boiled water.

Drink one cup, three times a day. If it's a real whopper of a headache, you can drink an additional three cups, six cups total, during the day.

b) Acute Killer Tincture — Add 10 drops each of tincture of hops (humulus) and tincture of scullcap (Scutellaria) into a glass of warm water.

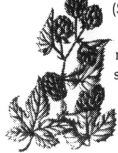

Drink one glass every 30 minutes, up to a maximum of six glasses. For the really daring, I suggest you put the tincture drops directly into the Acute Killer Tea. It packs a bigger punch.

Hops

Chronic Headaches

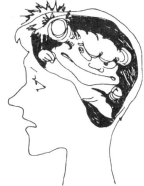

Unfortunately, there are headaches that won't go away. They recur with excru-ciating regularity. They are chronic, unrelenting, and for many, more than just a pain in the neck.

Usually, by the time I get to see patients with chronic headaches, they have already been to their family doctor. This is helpful. The doctor can help you zero-in on the cause of your headache while the natural medicine treatments described in this chapter can help alleviate or eliminate the root cause of your problem.

The following are the most likely causes of chronic headaches:

1. Migraine

Esther was only 11 years old when she came to see me. She had started getting terrible headaches together with nausea and vomiting. She had gone to the eye doctor who told her it was not related to her vision, which was 20/20. Her family doctor suggested she might be having migraines.

I asked Esther if she was under any sort of pressure. She said she didn't think so. But, when I asked her mother the same thing, she told me that Esther was the star pupil in her class and that the pressure to constantly be the best was becoming too much for her.

. "She sometimes stays up until 10:00 or 11:00 at night to finish a project," her mother complained. "If she doesn't get the best grades in class she gets very upset. She's a perfectionist."

Clearly, Esther was an obvious candidate for migraine headaches.

The Stress Factor

The most common symptoms of migraines are the following:

Flashes of light before eyes prior to the headache
Nausea or vomiting
Eyes become red and watery
Pain limited to one side of the head with the nostril on that
  side blocked

Migraine headaches tend to occur after days of accumulated stress. Teenagers are especially prone to headaches after school examinations, and perfectionists, like Esther, are the most prone to migraines.

Stress is a major factor in the cause of vasoconstriction, a squeezing of the tiny arteries in the head and eyes, which restricts blood supply to these areas.

The body then compensates with vasodilation, an expansion of the tiny blood vessels at the top of the head. This rapid dilating of blood vessels in the head is what produces the feeling of pain.

The Food Factor

Twenty-five percent of all migraines are caused by food allergies. Tyramine, a protein substance found in certain foods causes vasoconstriction. As we have seen above, this is the first step to migraine pain.

If you suspect you get migraine headaches, pay careful attention to the following foods which are high in tyramine. See if they may be causing your headaches:

> Chocolate
> Banana
> Avocado
> Yellow cheese
> Wine
> Raspberries

Aspartamine too, commonly used as an artificial sweetener, has been shown to trigger migraines in those susceptible to migraine headaches. Read food labels in order to avoid ingesting aspartamine.

Migraine Treatment

Don't panic at the first sign of a migraine attack or start feeling like an invalid. Jumping into bed may not be the best thing to do. All you can do there is focus on your pain.

Instead, begin winding down and try to distract yourself from the pain. Do light, easy activities and when your day is complete go to sleep, as usual.

If the pain is still throbbing inside your head, I suggest the following:

a. Try the methods mentioned earlier in this chapter for relief of acute headaches. They may work for the immediate pain you are experiencing. If they don't, then:

b. Take one day off to rest and relax. That's one day, not one week or one month. Missing too much school can put additional stress on you.

c. Eat only raw fruits and vegetables, and cooked vegetables for one day. Drink the juice of one ripe yellow lemon in water two-three times a day.

d. Take one capsule of vitamin E — 400 IU twice a day.

e. Take a Migraine-Killer Tincture: add 5 drops each of lavender, ginko biloba, feverfew, and scutellaria tinctures to a glass of warm water (a total of 20 drops). Drink one glass up to four times a day.

Feverfew

2. Hypoglycemia (low blood sugar)

One of the most common causes of headaches is a drop in blood sugar. This kind of headache tends to come a few hours after a meal, most often between 2:00 p.m. and 5:00 p.m., when the body is in its most alkaline chemical state. The drop in blood sugar and the alkaline state are both caused by a failure of the adrenal glands to secrete the adrenaline that raises low blood sugar.

Low Blood Sugar Treatment:

To fully understand the causes and effects of low blood sugar on your body, I suggest you read the section on low blood sugar in the chapter on fatigue. The main points to remember, however, are:

a) Eat small meals frequently instead of three big meals.

b) Support the adrenal glands with a vitamin B-complex supplement, from a rice source or food-grown source, one pill daily.

c) Take vitamin C — 500 mg. one pill twice a day with meals.

d) Stay clear of sugars and sweets.

3. Chinese Restaurant Syndrome

Chinese food is often loaded with a salt known as MSG (Monosodium Glutamate) which can cause headaches.

Avoid MSG. Many Chinese restaurants now offer their patrons the option of having food prepared without MSG. It

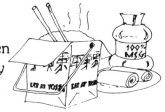

pays to ask. If you pick up a frozen Chinese dinner, read the label carefully to see if MSG has been used in preparing the meal.

4. Food Allergies And Sensitivities

It is no secret that allergic reactions to food can cause a number of unpleasant symptoms, including headaches. What you may not know is that some people may not experience an allergic reaction to the foods they eat until 24 hours later! This is called delayed food sensitivity.

If you are one of these people, trying to relate the cause of your headache to the foods you eat may be very difficult. Therefore, it is important to know what foods are the most likely to bring about headaches.

One recent study out of England known as the Egger Study found many common foods that cause headaches. The biggest culprit was regular cows' milk. Next came eggs followed by chocolate, wheat, cheese, and tomatoes.

The real surprise, however, was that children who suffered from headaches, and other discomfort, as a result of these foods, actually craved and ate a lot of the very foods which made them suffer.

If you suspect that you have a food allergy, see a specialist in Environmental Medicine. The doctor can help you determine whether you have food allergies or sensitivities.

In the meantime, try these supplements to help combat food sensitivities:

a. Vitamin C — 500 mg. one pill three times a day with meals.

b. Quercetin — one pill twice daily.

Hot Dog Headache

Hot dogs and salami are often treated with sodium nitrite or sodium nitrate. These preservatives have been shown to produce headaches in people who are sensitive to these chemicals.

5. Digestive-related Headache

If one or more of the secondary symptoms associated with your headache is heaviness in the abdomen, chronic gas, or constipation, then you may be able to treat your problem in a number of ways.

For best results, refer to the chapters in this book dealing with what are healthy foods and constipation. As you learn to purify your system, naturally, you will begin to get relief from your headaches.

6. Structural-related Headache

The spine and the neck are common targets of accumulated stress. Heavy lifting and minor injuries can move the spinal vertebrae out of line from their natural position. Headaches are often related to problems of the neck vertebrae and tensions in the neck muscles.

Chiropractic Treatment

Structural headaches are often helped by a visit (or a series of visits) to your local chiropractor. Chiropractors are highly trained therapists who work with their hands to correct problems of the back and neck. They are not medical doctors. However, all chiropractors receive a four-five year medical education before beginning their practice.

Chiropractic therapy has advanced tremendously over the past 30 years. I have referred many cases of chronic headaches to chiropractors who treat the skull itself with cranial therapy. This therapy offers diagnosis and treatment of long-forgotten childhood bumps and bangs to the head which can cause headaches 10 years down the road.

When asked to sum up the goal of the chiropractic treatment, one practitioner responded, "When your spine is in line you feel fine."

7. Dental-related Headache

Some people get headaches soon after a visit to the dentist. At first glance that's hard to believe since much of dentistry today is painless and you don't actually feel the drilling. But what the dentist does may exert a lot of stress upon the bones of the face and jaw, particularly the temporo-mandibular joint (TMJ).

TMJ Treatment

If you feel that your headaches are related to dental treatments, see a chiropractor. Many of them are specially trained in the diagnosis and correction of TMJ syndrome. Call and ask if your local chiropractor has TMJ training. Correction of the TMJ is a simple, painless procedure.

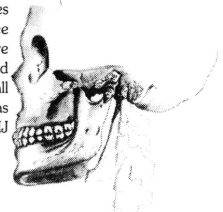

8. Sinusitis-related Headache

Sinusitis is an infection of the sinuses. When the sinuses fill with mucous, pressure can build up. With or without infection this pressure can cause a dull nagging headache.

Headaches that tend to appear above one eye only may be related to sinusitis.

Sinusitis Headache Treatment

a) Cut out all milk products, egg whites and white flour.

b) Take vitamin C — 500 mg. one pill three times a day.

c) Try a salt water nasal flush — Mix one teaspoon of salt with 3/4 cup warm water. Put eight droppers full of the solution into each nostril, once a day. Allow the solution to run out of your nose into a tissue between each dropper full.

9. Menstrual-related Headache

One of the most common forms of headache in young women occurs either before or during the menstrual period. The full range of symptoms associated with menstruation is dealt with in the chapter called PMS. Both the raspberry leaf tea and vitamin B-6 mentioned in that chapter should bring you relief if you suffer from menstrual-related headaches.

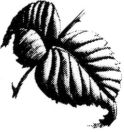

Raspberry leaf

10. Eyestrain

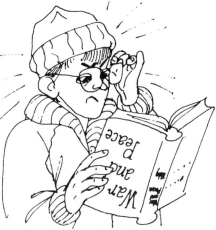

Poorly fitted glasses, an improper lens prescription, or not wearing glasses when you actually need them can cause eyestrain headache. Nausea, as a result of prolonged reading, is a classic sign of headache related to visual problems.

The best solution to eyestrain headache is to get an eye examination and follow the optometrist's advice.

11. Oxygen Deficiency

Lack of oxygen may be the cause of your headaches. If you find you are dizzy walking up stairs or are constantly opening the window to get more air, you probably lack oxygen.

These symptoms may indicate anemia, the deficiency of hemoglobin, due to a lack of red blood cells in the blood. The red blood cells transport oxygen and other nutrients to all the cells of the body. If your red blood count is low, less oxygen than normal is being sent to the different parts of your body. Your body signals its distress by giving you a headache or making you dizzy after only a little exertion.

Anemia Treatment

Have your doctor test you for anemia. If you are anemic, follow the relevant advice given in the chapter on fatigue.

Not all people who are oxygen-deficient suffer from anemia.

Other indications of oxygen deficiency include:

Black and blue marks after the slightest bump

Constantly red lines on the whites of the eye

Bleeding gums

In any case of suspected oxygen deficiency, you should:

a. Exercise in the open air.

b. Take vitamin E — 400 IU twice daily.

c. Take vitamin C — 500 mg. with bioflavonoids, twice daily.

Chapter Six

Weight Loss

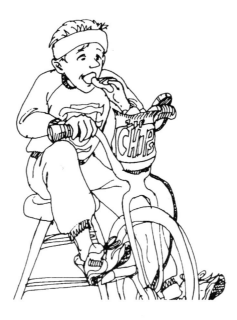

These days I see a parade of young girls, between the ages of 14 and 17, coming into my office, weighing about 80 pounds, wearing a size four dress, and asking me to help them lose that "extra five pounds." Too often, I find that these girls have developed an obsessive need to keep losing weight, no matter how thin they are. Some of them have all the symptoms of anorexia, and I usually refer them (and their parents) to a psychologist.

For most teens between the ages of 14 and 17, 75 pounds is not a realistic goal weight. Nor should it be. Depending on age and height, neither may 85, 95, or even 105 pounds, for that matter.

Obviously, ideal weights vary (see chart below). Nevertheless, your overall state of health plays an important role in determining what kind of weight goal you set for yourself.

The Correct Approach To Weight Loss

Weight loss diets are so popular these days it seems that there are more diets than dieters. And still we see that many people fail to lose weight, while others tend to yo-yo (lose-gain-lose-gain).

Part of the problem with slimming diets is that they force you to concentrate on calories, rather then on healthy living.

It's true that if you drink a 250-calorie milk shake loaded with vitamins and minerals twice a day, you can lose weight...and fast. But it is also true that, in the long run, not all the vitamins and minerals they contain are good for you. And, you can't drink these shakes forever. Inevitably, before too long, the weight comes rolling back.

My approach to weight loss centers around the following two key points:

1. You should never sacrifice good health in order to lose weight.

2. While losing weight you should actually be building your general health.

Are You Overweight?

Has anyone ever said to you:

"You know why you're out of breath? Because you're fat!"

or,

"That's a really cute double chin you're growing there."

or,

" Your stomach got here 10 minutes before you did."

I encounter many teens who are emotionally scarred because they were always known as "the fat kid," or were the butt of jokes by their classmates. By the time they enter my office they have tried half-a-dozen diets, all to no avail. What they need is direction, and a clear understanding of what being overweight means. The first thing you should know about being overweight is what that means:

Overweight is weight that exceeds the standard ideal weight set according to body size, height, exercise and lifestyle. Obesity is defined as 20 percent more than the established ideal weight.

That means that until you are 20 percent more than your ideal weight, you are overweight, not obese. You should watch your weight, not panic and certainly not crash diet. Rather, begin by setting a realistic weight-loss goal.

Use the following chart to determine your approximate ideal weight.

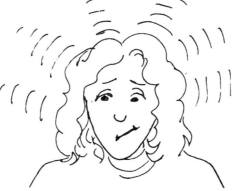

Don't Panic!

Standard Weights According To Height and Age:

Male:

Age	Average Height	Range	Average Weight	Range
11	57"	(52"- 62")	77 lbs.	(59-113)
12	60	(55"- 64")	87	(66-128)
13	63	(57"- 68")	99	(74-143)
14	65	(60"- 71")	111	(84-159)
15	68	(62"- 73")	125	(95-174)
16	70	(64"- 74")	137	(105-188)
17	71	(66"- 75")	146	(113-200)
18	71	(67"- 76")	152	(118-210)

Female:

Age	Average Height	Range	Average Weight	Range
11	55"	(51"- 62")	81 lbs.	(60-118)
12	61	(56"- 65")	91	(67-133)
13	63	(58"- 67")	101	(75-148)
14	64	(59"- 68")	110	(83-160)
15	65	(61"- 69")	118	(90-171)
16	65	(61"- 69")	122	(95-178)
17	65	(61"- 69")	125	(98-181)
18	65	(61"- 69")	125	(99-181)

How To Set Up A Workable Weight Loss Program

Any weight loss program must take into account the following points:

Adequate Nutrition

Eating less calories will surely help to take off inches, but as the calories decrease so do your chances of achieving adequate nutrition. If you eat less than 1000 calories per day, you cannot obtain all the nutrition set forth by the RDA (Recommended Dietary Allowance).

Therefore, don't risk your health in order to lose weight!

Lifestyle Changes

In order to change your diet you may need to change your lifestyle. You can do it, it's not so hard. Plan to meet your friends at the salad bar instead of the pizza parlor. Break the coffee and cake habit in the morning, and eat some oatmeal instead.

Enjoy Your Diet

The more you eat whole natural foods, the more your taste buds adapt. Soon you will lose your craving for salt, sweets and rich foods.

The ideal diet should become part of your lifestyle, not a burden imposed upon you. That's important! The new, healthy foods must appeal to you even after the inches come off. That way you'll continue eating correctly and won't put back on those extra pounds.'

That "Full" Feeling

Your mother is right. You should chew your food well. Chewing properly sets in action a string of chemical reactions that enable your brain to determine exactly when your body is satisfied. If you gulp down your food without chewing well, you can end up eating two or three times more food than you need. That's a lot of extra calories!

Eat foods high in fiber such as raw salads and wheat bran. The fiber expands inside your stomach and gives you a feeling of fullness.

Finally, include some protein in your meals in order to prolong the time it takes the stomach to empty. Protein provides a feeling of fullness while fulfilling an important dietary requirement. Examples of healthy proteins include: fish, chicken, turkey, soya tofu and lentils.

The Down Side of Dieting

There are dangers and pitfalls you should be aware of when you choose a weight loss program.

The rule of thumb is: Never jeopardize your health.

Don't Take Drugs Or Chemicals

Diet should not be based on drugs or chemicals. You should never take amphetamines ("speed") which cause the metabolism to speed up. At the end of the artificial "high," caused by the drug, the metabolism becomes more sluggish than when you began and you rapidly gain back the lost weight.

There are diet doctors who prescribe amphetamines. My advice to you: Stay away from them!

Drugs and losing weight don't mix, not in the long run. Not if you want the weight to stay off...permanently.

Pass The Carbohydrates, Please

While giving up carbohydrates like sugar, cakes, sodas and chocolate harms no one but the sugar manufacturers, there are natural carbohydrates that contribute to good health as well as help prevent disease.

Examples of healthy carbohydrates, which should be part of your weight-loss program, include vegetables like pumpkin, carrots, celery root, parsley root, artichoke, zucchini and other squashes. Cooked grains like brown rice, buckwheat or millet and other complex carbohydrates are essential for your diet program.

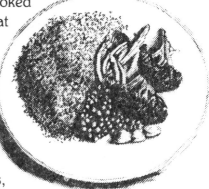

If you cut out all carbohydrates, fruits, vegetables, potatoes and legumes from your diet, you will deprive yourself of precious vitamins, minerals and fiber.

Worse still, if your body is deprived completely of the carbohydrates it needs for energy, it will eventually begin to break down the fat reserves in your body and, in certain cases, release substances called "ketones." These are extremely acidic and toxic, usually causing nausea and breathing problems.

Therefore including some healthy carbohydrates in your diet will cancel out this potential problem.

The Protein Problem

Your diet should not contain massive amounts of protein.

Most dieters instinctively cut down on carbohydrates and increase their protein intake. The fact is, many weight loss programs recommend high protein intake.

This appeals to the average dieter because protein usually tastes good and is filling. But watch out! Here are some good reasons to be careful about how much protein you consume.

a) The liver and kidneys are the organs that bear the burden of excess protein. Nitrogen compounds such as uric acid result from the normal breakdown of dietary proteins. Too much protein produces an excess of nitrogen. Excess nitrogen cannot be eliminated by the liver and kidneys and accumulates in the body. It has been shown that this nitrogen accumulation can cause arthritis, heart disease, kidney disease and even cancer.

b) Undigested, excess proteins can accumulate in the intestines causing constipation, gas and (phew!) chronic bad breath.

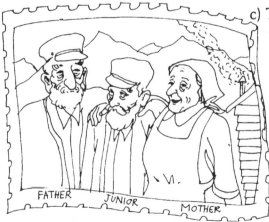

FATHER   JUNIOR   MOTHER

c) The life expectancy of people who have a relatively low protein intake is considerably longer than those who have a high protein diet. For example, many of the inhabitants of Hunza, Bulgaria, Russia and the Yucatan are still going strong, well into their 90s, on a very low animal protein diet (approximately 25 grams per day).

d) Excess protein intake can lead to deficiencies of vitamins B-3, B-6, and magnesium. These nutrients are essential for proper brain function. Furthermore, the high phosphorous content of animal proteins may lead to calcium deficiency.

How Much Protein Is Too Much?

I believe that the maximum amount of protein for a person seeking to lose weight should be approximately 1 gram of protein for every 2.2 lbs. of body weight. Consult the following chart to find out how much daily protein that means for you:

Your current weight in pounds	Maximum daily protein intake
100	.45 grams
110	.50 grams
120	.55 grams
130	.60 grams
140	.64 grams
150	.68 grams
160	.72 grams
180	.81 grams

To understand this better, let's take a look at some of the proteins an average dieter may eat during the course of the day.

Breakfast
8-ounce glass of milk =	8 grams of protein.
2 eggs =	12 grams protein

Lunch
2 tablespoons of protein powder in a glass of milk =	38 grams of protein

Supper
6-ounce steak =	35 grams of protein

GRAND TOTAL = 93 grams of protein

Unless you weigh over 200 pounds, this is way too much protein. And almost one-third of it comes from the protein powder in milk that you are taking to lose weight.

Here's Why You Gain Weight

1. Insufficient Exercise

For most people losing weight means eating less. And, at first glance, that does seem to be the case.

For example: If you eat 500 calories less each day of the week, at the end of the week you will have lost 3,500 calories (500 x 7 = 3,500).

Sounds like a lot doesn't it? But 3,500 calories equals only one pound! And it takes an awful lot of willpower to refuse 3,500 calories of junkfood a week. So the only logical thing to do is to add exercise to your diet.

For example, 30 minutes of brisk walking burns at least 150 calories of energy expenditure. If you jogged for 30 minutes a day every day of the week, the calories burned would equal 7 x 150 = 1050 calories. If you continued to jog like this for 10 weeks you would burn off 1050 x 10 = 10,500 calories, or three pounds.

With a pair of headphones and a treadmill, half-an-hour of jogging a day should be a breeze. The important thing to remember is that in order to get rid of your fat you must exercise.

But not all exercises get rid of all fat. There is a major difference between body fat and muscle fat.

As we grow out of our active childhood the body begins depositing a higher percentage of fat within the muscle tissue. Adult muscle tissue is composed of 12-22 percent muscle fat. Athletes have much less fat in their muscles, about 5-6 percent. When the fat within the muscle is higher than it should be you become not merely overweight, but "overfat."

While normal weight-loss diets will reduce fat stores or "overweight," few diets will truly reduce the excess fat within the muscle tissue. The only way to burn off muscle fat is through aerobic exercise.

Aerobic exercise can be almost any activity that you perform non-stop for a minimum of 10 minutes — and which causes you to breathe more quickly. This may include dancing, skipping rope, bicycle riding, running, and swimming. (Never swim in cold water, because the cold tells the brain to store fat for heat insulation.)

Below is an activity chart to help you decide which exercises are best for you, and which bring you the quickest weight loss.

NUMBER OF CALORIES BURNED IN 10 MINUTES ACCORDING TO YOUR BODY WEIGHT.

if you weigh

ACTIVITY	125 LBS.	150 LBS.	175 LBS.
Baseball	39	47	54
Basketball	58	70	82
Dancing (moderate)	35	42	48
Football	69	83	96
Golfing	33	40	48
Racquetball/squash	75	90	104
Skiing	80	96	112
Swimming, crawl (20 yards/min)	40	48	56
Tennis	56	67	80
Volleyball	43	52	65

2. Constant Hunger

Are you always hungry?

You may have an inefficient digestive system, which can cause you to gain weight. This condition can occur due to any number of things including overeating, poor food combinations, physical problems or genetic makeup. As a result, you can be constantly hungry despite that fact that you eat enough, or more than enough, food.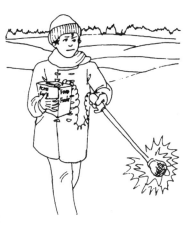

Check with your doctor. If you are hungry because you have an inability to process your food — weak stomach acids, insufficient pancreatic enzymes — then try the following digestive enzymes.

a) Apple cider vinegar — one teaspoon in a glass of water before protein-rich meals (meats, fish, eggs, beans, etc.) will aid protein digestion.

b) Bromelain — 100 mg. one pill after meals, twice daily, aids starch digestion (bread, potatoes, rice, etc.).

3. Wacky Appestat

The appestat is the brain control center of the appetite. It tells you when you are hungry and when you are full. When it is out-of-whack you may be getting the wrong signals. You may find yourself feeling hungry when you just ate a big meal.

A wacky appestat can be triggered by:

a) Low blood sugar (hypoglycemia). The brain requires sugar in order to keep functioning. In the absence of blood sugar the appestat will increase the urge to eat.

b) High blood sugar (diabetes). Diabetics have high blood sugar by definition, yet they cannot get this sugar into their deprived and hungry cells for two reasons:

  1) Diabetics often have high blood fats, which physically inhibit the sugar from getting where it needs to go.

  2) They may also have mineral deficiencies (such as zinc or chromium) which also inhibit the natural cellular use of sugar.

  Once again, in the absence of fuel (sugar) on a cellular level, the appestat will increase hunger.

The Natural Way To Reduce Appetite

Use Those Teeth!

Chew every mouthful at least 50 times. Chewing allows for maximum breakdown of food and gives the appestat time to truly determine the amount of food you need to feel satisfied.

Ear Acupuncture

Ouch! If you are afraid of needles, raise your hand.

In the hands of a trained acupuncturist, you will barely — if at all — feel those needles.

Acupuncture needles applied to the ears have gained much public attention over the past 10 years. Almost everyone knows someone who claims that ear acupuncture has helped them successfully reduce their appetite or overcome a smoking habit.

Bulking Agents

Natural bulking agents fill up the stomach and inform the brain that you've eaten enough. They help you to eat less food but still feel satisfied. The following bulking agents help give you that "full" feeling and should be eaten five minutes before each meal:

Raw bran — one tablespoon in a glass of water.

Alfalfa tablets — 500 mg. Chew one tablet immediately before meals.

Natural Appetite Suppressors

Spirulina — 225 mg. one tablet two times a day before meals.

Apple cider vinegar — one teaspoon in a glass of water before a protein meal such as meat, chicken, fish, eggs, or beans.

Your Last Weight-loss Program

If you follow my easy-to-use weight-loss program you won't have to suck in your gut to put on those pants you bought just two months ago. Nor will you have to move out that button on your skirt, again.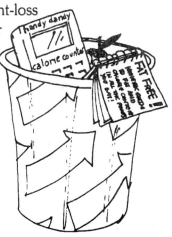

Best of all, six months from now — unless you grow out of them — your clothes will still fit you around the waist...and everywhere else.

Oh yes, you can put away those

pocket calorie counters. You're better off spending your time chewing. Just follow this diet plan, like hundreds of other teens have done over the years, and you will lose pounds and stay healthy.

Choose only one option for each meal:

Early Morning "Wake-up"

One tall glass of water with one teaspoon of apple cider vinegar.

One tall glass of water with one tablespoon of freshly squeezed lemon juice (from ripe yellow lemons only).

Breakfast

If it's a school day and you're in a rush, eat one grapefruit or two medium size non-sweet apples (Granny or Jonathan).

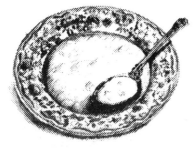 If you have the time, eat a natural grain cereal. Rye cereal is the best. Millet porridge is second and oatmeal is your third choice. Whichever you choose, add one heaping tablespoon of wheat bran or oat bran to the cereal.

For a change of pace, try a small can of water-packed tuna fish with a large green salad.

Lunch

Large green salad topped with low-fat cottage cheese.

Bowl of brown rice or kasha (buckwheat) with cooked

vegetables (zucchini, green beans, cabbage, cauliflower, carrots, onions, etc).

Mid-afternoon Snack

One glass of water with one teaspoon of apple cider vinegar.

One glass of carrot-celery juice (50/50).

One glass of bottled pomegranate juice mixed with water (75 percent juice and 25 percent water).

Dinner

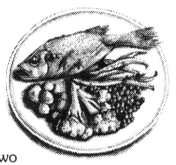

Baked fish or chicken with any cooked vegetables (except potatoes, sweet potatoes and eggplant).

Fish has the upper hand over poultry because it contains two substances which actually encourage weight loss: fish oils reduce blood cholesterol and iodine which stimulates the thyroid gland which, in turn, speeds up your metabolism.

Tofu (soya cheese) with cooked vegetables.

Thick lentil soup with cooked vegetables.

Late-night snack

Popcorn prepared without oil
Carrot sticks
Celery sticks
Rice cakes

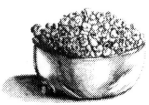

And That's Not All!

Here are some additional foods that will enrich your diet without making you go off it. You can add these to your diet or substitute them for one of the snacks.

Choose two or three of the following every day:

Potassium broth: Make this soup from well-scrubbed potato peels and carrots. Have as much as you want!

Seaweed broth: Add one strip of kombu (or any other seaweed) to any soup.

Sprouts. Eat as much as you want!

Low-calorie fruit is a healthy treat. Enjoy tart apples, pomegranate, grapefruit or pomelo.

Natural Medicines That Help You Lose Weight

Sometimes a person's "will" is not equal to his "power." You may really want to get on the weight-loss program, but after a day or two, well, you go back to your old ways. You may not have the staying power to follow through with the program.

Why this happens is hard to say. However, one thing is sure. You have to be psyched-up to start a weight-loss program and you have to maintain that level of interest for quite some time. If you're not ready then no one can convince you.

But don't give up! Natural medicines can help you lose weight. And once you get started, who knows, you may get that will-power you've been missing, to reach your weight loss goal.

Here's what I recommend:

Lecithin — 1200 mg. one capsule daily with meals. Lecithin lowers fat and cholesterol levels in the blood.

Glucomannan — one capsule twice daily before meals. It provides some of the best plant fiber prescribed for weight-loss diets.

Spirulina — 300 mg. two tablets twice daily either with meals or between meals. Spirulina is a blue-green algae that offers perhaps the largest spectrum of vitamins, minerals and trace elements available in one natural food.

Bromelain — 100 mg. one pill daily after starchy foods such as bread, potatoes, rice, etc. Bromelaine is a pineapple enzyme that breaks down starch in foods.

Cornsilk tea — one tablespoon steeped in one cup of boiled water. Drink one cup twice a day between meals. This is a natural diuretic to remove excess water from the body.

Chapter Seven
Allergies, Colds & Viruses

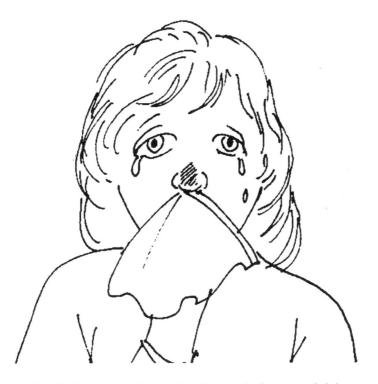

In the "olden days" people depended an awful lot on a combination of healthy foods and medicinal plants to prevent and cure everything from the common cold to meningitis and heart disease.

Needless to say, just because the cures were natural was no guarantee they would be effective. The fact is, that while many diseases were indeed cured by home-grown remedies, many other diseases could not be. Their elimination came about with the discovery of antibiotics.

The Antibiotic Dilemma

Antibiotics are certainly wonder drugs. They help the body get rid of "foreign" invaders like nasty germs and bacteria. But they present a host of problems as well.

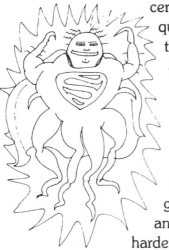

The bacteria that invade your system may be killed by a certain antibiotic but, as science is quickly discovering, the few bacteria that survive become immune to that antibiotic. This hardier, stronger bacteria needs yet another antibiotic to kill it. And still some survive. Which demands a new antibiotic which does not kill all the bacteria... You get the picture. The cycle goes on and on. We are always trying to get one step ahead of the mutating and evolving bacteria. But it's getting harder and harder.

Antibiotics are not picky. They end up destroying all the bacteria, both bad and good, in your intestinal tract. This can cause constipation and chronic gas.

When young children take repeated courses of antibiotic treatment at an early age, their immature immune systems do not produce the quantity and quality of antibodies necessary to ward off disease on their own. The antibiotics do all the work, and the children become dependent on them. Their immune systems do not develop properly, leaving the children open to a variety of infections.

And finally, while antibiotics destroy germs, germs are not necessarily what cause disease and infection. Germs are a result of the disease process. They are symptoms of some other, more basic, problem within the body. When the body has been weakened by poor nutrition, excessive stress, insufficient sleep, or other problems, your immune system doesn't work properly and you are much more susceptible to infection and disease. Using antibiotics to destroy the germs is only half the answer. You have to create a healthy body so that germs won't be able to harm your system in the first place.

The best way for you to stay healthy and thus limit the use of antibiotics is to eat properly, exercise regularly and get adequate sleep. This will build up the natural defenses of your immune system.

The Body's Defenses

When you have symptoms of a cold, virus or flu it means your body is trying to get rid of the invading germ by itself. And that's good. Here's a short list of what your body does, and why:

1) Swollen glands are a sign that your body is busy destroying all kinds of "invaders" and foreign proteins. The harder they work for you, the more your glands swell up.

2) A high fever means that your body is heating itself up to kill the "invader." Obviously, your body can't heat up too high or it will damage your vital organs. That's why we try to bring a fever down when it gets too high (see below).

3) Mucous, and a runny nose, are the body's way of flushing out the "invaders" and lubricating irritated nasal passages.

"Bug" Busters

At the first sign of a cold, virus or flu attack, try this natural treatment (do all these steps):

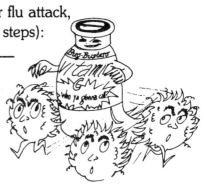

1. Vitamin C (with bioflavonoids) — 1000 mg. one pill twice a day.

2. Beta-carotene — 10,000 IU one capsule two times a day.

3. Garlic — 500 mg. two capsules three times a day.

4. Propolis tincture — 15 drops twice a day.

5. Rosemary and thyme herbal tea — Boil three cups of water. Add three teaspoons each of rosemary and thyme. Steep for five minutes. Strain. Divide into three cups. Drink one cup three times a day.

6. Eat only raw fruits and cooked vegetables the whole day.

7. Echinacea root — 400 mg. two capsules twice a day.

8. Drink. Drink. Drink.

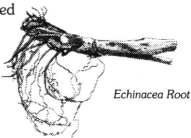

Echinacea Root

Follow this treatment for at least two days. If the cold, virus or flu hits you anyhow, you should find that your body has an easier time fighting off the lingering effects.

Fever Tactics

Fever is the body's response to an invasion of bacteria. It heats itself up to kill the bacteria that are feeding on waste products in the body. By reducing the waste products in the body you help to eliminate the need for fever.

When fever strikes, it's best to fast for a day, drinking only teas, juices and water. If you are really hungry, have a bowl of onion soup two to three times throughout the day. Onion soup produces an immediate sweat which will help to cool the body and remove toxins.

And try these other remedies to help cool a fever, naturally:

1. Rub your body with a warm cloth soaked in water and apple cider vinegar.

2. Drink ginger tea — 1/4 teaspoon of ginger powder in one cup of boiled water. Or, drink linden flower tea — one tablespoon of linden flower in a cup of boiled water.

Sore Throat Relief

For natural relief from a sore throat try one of the following:

1. Zinc gluconate lozenges — 22 mg. one lozenge twice a day.
2. Licorice root tincture — 25 drops twice a day.
3. Propolis drops — 15 drops twice a day.
4. Warm salt water gargle — one teaspoon of salt in a cup of water (gargle but do not swallow).

What is An Allergy?

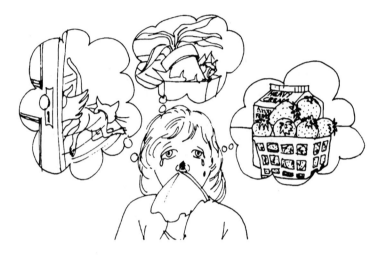

Do you suffer from any of the following symptoms?

Reddening of the skin

Sneezing attacks

Breathing difficulties

Your problem may be allergies.

Most people spend a lot of time and money trying to identify what they are allergic to, and then avoid those things like the plague.

Allergic to cats? Get rid of your cat. Allergic to food? Get rid of the food. Allergic to plants? Get rid of the plant. Allergic to teachers? Get rid of...

At the end of the day many people have gotten rid of everything and still feel sick. So, they pack up and head for Arizona where the dry weather seems to help.

I'm not too keen on the "get rid of it" approach. I prefer to attack allergies at a·cellular level.

On the cellular level, antibodies located at the mouth, nose and throat wait to latch onto and destroy foreign "invaders." When bacteria or pollens enter the body they are attracted to the antibodies which sit on the surface of special mast cells. A battle ensues between the invader and the anti-bodies. In the course of the struggle, irritation is produced on the mast cells causing them to explode. The explosion releases histamine and other chemicals from inside the mast cells, producing the unpleasant symptoms of allergies.

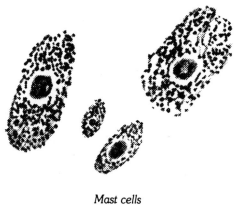

Mast cells

Hoẅ To̊ Fig̊ht *Allergies*

If we could stop the mast cells from bursting we would prevent the symptoms of allergy. Here are a group of nutrients that help stabilize cell membranes and give structural support to cells.

Take this group of five supplements for one month, at those times of year when your allergies flare up.

1. Calcium Ascorbate — combines 50 mg. calcium and 500 mg. vitamin C. One pill three times a day.
2. Citrus biofalvonoids — 1000 mg. one pill twice a day.
3. Quercetin-C — 250 mg. one pill twice a day.

4. Vitamin B-5 (pantothenic acid) — 100 mg. one pill twice a day.

5. Licorice root tincture — 20 drops twice a day.

A Fungus Among Us

Fungus is an equal opportunity attacker, with teens a common host. And fungus grows both on our bodies and inside our intestinal tract.

The most common form of fungus is called candida. Actually, candida is a natural organism of the body. However, for a variety of reasons — too much sugar or starch in your diet, too much alcohol, sensitivities to foods containing yeast, allergies to molds — candida suddenly changes its structure, increases in number and becomes invasive and aggressive, creating many symptoms such as:

Athlete's foot

Yeast infections

Intestinal gas

Food allergies

General fatigue

Fungus Busters

If you have any of the above symptoms of candidal growth, then you should eliminate sugar, alcohol and yeast products from your diet because these are the primary fuels for candida growth. Also avoid damp and moldy places.

To help your immune system fight the fungal growth, here is a regimen that has proven effective for many teens I've treated for fungal infections. Take all five of the following supplements for one month and see if it helps:

1. Liquid garlic — 50 drops three times a day.
2. Caprylic acid pills — 100 mg. one pill twice a day.
3. Vitamin C — 500 mg. one pill three times a day.
4. Acidophilus pills — one pill three times a day.
5. Biotin — 400 micrograms once a day.

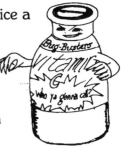

Cold Sores

Cold sores, also called canker sores or fever blisters, are caused by the Herpes Simplex virus. This virus affects millions of us. In about 90 percent of the population it lies dormant, never causing an outbreak of these painful blisters. But if you are in the other 10 percent, you know the burning and stinging pain these small red dots that turn into blisters in and around your mouth can cause.

Nobody knows, for sure, what causes these outbreaks but there are various factors that seem to bring them on, including:

Allergies to most nuts, avocado, chocolate and gelatin
Stress
Sunburn (another kind of stress)

It's best to avoid these, if possible. Use the following treatment chart to determine which supplements can be useful to either treat an active outbreak of sores, or to be used as a preventive measure to avoid an outbreak.

Cold Sore Treatment/Prevention

Supplement	Preventive Dose	Outbreak Treatment
Zinc Picolinate 15 mg.	Once a day	Three times a day
Vitamin C 500 mg.	Three times a day	Two pills, twice a day
Acidophilus capsules	Once a day	Two capsules, three times a day
Beta-carotene 25,000 IU	Once a day	Twice a day
Lysine 500 mg.	Once a day	Three times a day

Two of the 26 amino acids have been found to be related to the Herpes Simplex virus. An excess of arginine and/or deficiency of lysine can be fuel for a herpes outbreak.

Reduce Arginine Foods	Increase Lysine Foods
Chocolate	Turkey
Peanuts	Chicken
Brazil nuts	Halibut fish
Almonds	Tuna fish
Sesame seeds	

Chapter Eight

PMS

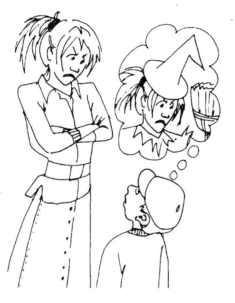

Many teenage girls experience discomfort, usually before and/or during their menstrual period. Various aches and pains are common, although not experienced by everyone. The most common symptoms include:

Cramps in the lower abdomen

Low back pain

Nausea and/or vomiting

Emotional instability including anxiety, irritability, depression and crying spells

Headaches

Fatigue

Bloating

When these symptoms occur the week before your menstrual flow begins, these symptoms are called Premenstrual Syndrome, or PMS. When they occur during your flow, they are called Dysmenorrhea or difficult menstruation.

These aches and pains are due to hormonal changes related to the menstrual process. It can take a year or so for a young woman's reproductive system to mature fully after menstruation begins. Even after the first year some young women continue to suffer from symptoms.

Sima

Sima was just 12 when she had her first period. The discomfort, headaches and irritability she felt for about a week before the onset of her menstrual flow lessened considerably as soon as she began bleeding. Her mother told her that her experience was natural for girls who were having their period for the first time.

"I'm 14 now and, if anything, the pain and discomfort are worse," Sima confided. "I get these terrible mood swings and then about two days before I start bleeding I get so depressed I can't say a nice word to anyone. I can't stand myself then. I feel bloated, gaseous and miserable."

Debra

Debra came to my office with her mother. She was 15 but looked much older. She appeared to be very tired and was having trouble sitting still.

"Debra gets like this every month now," her mother told me. "She didn't have any problems with her period until about half a year ago. Then she started complaining of headaches. She can't sleep. She's fidgety. And if her siblings even look at her the wrong way she starts screaming.

"What can we do? Our family doctor told us she'll just have to learn to cope. The problem is the rest of us can't cope with her moodiness. Yesterday my youngest came back from school and asked me if the witch was home."

Both Sima and Debra got relief from their symptoms by following the steps outlined below.

Hormonal Imbalances

No one has proven conclusively what causes PMS but most theories point to hormonal imbalances involving the female hormones estrogen and progesterone.

Several studies have found that, at this time, young women who suffer from PMS, have hormonal levels that vary considerably from the norm.

Adrenal Glands

It may be that your blood sugar or blood pressure drops just before your period begins. If so, it is a case of adrenal gland insufficiency and probably contributes to the fatigue you feel at this time.

The adrenal glands secrete hormones that raise the blood sugar and elevate blood pressure. When they are not functioning up to par, you will feel listless and tired.

Food cravings, the sudden "need" to eat starches and sweets, are also a symptom of PMS, specifically adrenal insufficiency. If the adrenals do not help the body keep its sugar level stable, the drop in sugar will signal your brain to "crave" sugar.

Included in the treatment below you will find suggestions on how to keep your blood sugar stable, which many of my patients tell me greatly reduces their feeling of fatigue.

Nine Proven Steps to Prevention/Treatment of PMS

This is a well-integrated natural health plan designed to prevent or alleviate your PMS. Follow all the steps every day, beginning one week before the start of your menstrual flow and continue until the symptoms subside.

1. Take Calcium-magnesium Supplements

Excellent research exists to verify that calcium reduces the pain and discomfort of PMS. Natural medicine views the mineral magnesium as the natural tranquilizer of the human body. Together, these two minerals form a very efficient barrier against many of the symptoms of PMS. Calcium should be taken with its partner magnesium in the ratio of two parts calcium to one part magnesium:

Calcium carbonate — 500 mg. and magnesium - 250 mg. twice a day with meals.

2. Include Foods High In Calcium And Magnesium In Your Diet

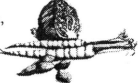

a) High calcium foods: sesame tahina, almonds, carrots, cabbage, soya milk, tofu (ready-made soya bean cheese).

b) High magnesium foods: dried figs and prunes, cooked cereal of ground yellow corn meal, whole-grain breakfast cereal, romaine lettuce.

3. The Vitamin Connection

Vitamin B-6 works well with magnesium in the war against PMS. This vitamin has proven to be a most trusted friend assuming one does not overdo a good thing. That means, stick to the recommended dose:

Vitamin B-6 — 50 mg. one tablet twice a day with meals.

4. Watch Your Sugar Intake

a) Keep your blood sugar level up by avoiding sweets. The more sugar you eat the more insulin your pancreas secretes. Insulin gets sugar out of the blood very quickly. This sudden removal of sugar can cause headaches, dizziness and disorientation. Just about the last thing you need during your period.

b) Include high protein foods (chicken, fish, eggs) in your diet. Protein helps stabilize blood sugar levels. For a complete understanding read the section on low blood sugar in the fatigue chapter.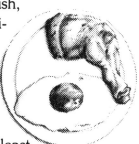

c) Eat smaller meals more frequently, at least four-five small meals per day. This keeps you from gorging on sweets or other foods that are not good for you. It also helps you control those food cravings.

5. Evening Primrose Oil

The fatty acid called gama-linoleic acid is found concentrated in a plant oil called Evening Primrose. It helps to regulate most menstrual problems, especially any form of breast swelling or discomfort. Unfortunately, your body does not get enough of this fatty acid from the foods you eat.

Take evening primrose oil capsules — 500 mg. one capsule three times a day, with meals.

6. The Nut Connection

Many of my patients report that they crave nuts and seeds particularly during their menstrual cycle. Almonds, sunflower seeds, pumpkin seeds, sesame seeds and sesame seed tahina are rich sources of natural fats and the mineral zinc. Your body needs these nutrients to help regulate your hormones.

7. Tea Time

a) Raspberry leaf has been called "The Woman's Herb" because of its overall medicinal effect on women's cycles. I advise my patients to drink one cup of raspberry leaf tea three times a day, between meals.

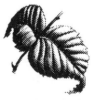

How to prepare: Add one full tablespoon of raspberry leaves to a cup of boiled water. Let it soak for four minutes. Sweeten with a teaspoon of honey.

Raspberry leaf

b) For many girls bloating is the worst effect of their period. They report feeling sluggish and nauseous. If water retention is one of your problems, try this sure-fire tea. It's best to drink one cup three times a day, between meals.

How to prepare: Add one tablespoon of cornsilk and one teaspoon of dried parsley to a cup of boiled water. Let it soak for four minutes.

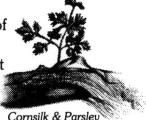

Cornsilk & Parsley

8. Anti-cramping Tincture

This mixture will help to relieve symptoms of the lower abdominal cramping and lower back pain that can result from PMS:

Crampbark (viburnum opulis) 15 drops

Skullcap (scutellaria) 15 drops

Drink 2-3 times daily in water or herbal tea.

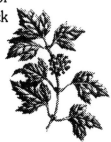

Crampbark

9. Yoga, Stretching, & Exercise

It's probably the last thing you want to hear when you're feeling bloated and uncomfortable, but a regimen of exercise definitely reduces tension. When you are more relaxed your body works more efficiently. You feel more limber, and can usually control your discomfort better.

Chapter Nine

Fatigue

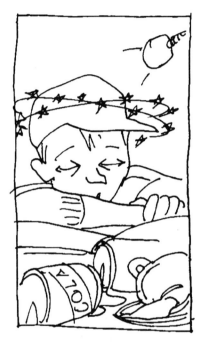

"I'm really tired lately," Rachel sighed. "My get up and go just got up and went one day. I barely even have the strength to go from class to class in school."

"How long have you been feeling like this?" I asked her.

"It seems like forever, but I guess it's only been since I started gaining weight. Everyone said that maybe I was tired because I was so thin. I started eating more because I thought it would give me more energy. But it's just the opposite! Now I feel fat...and even more tired."

Fatigue is the most common complaint I hear these days. It spans all age groups, but while older people come in to get something to give them a "pick-me-up," teens usually feel they are going through some phase that will pass. It rarely does.

Let's take a look at some of the basic causes of fatigue:

1. Constipation

You must have a bowel movement every day. The accumulated wastes in the colon produce toxins, gas, and unhealthy bacteria that leave you feeling sluggish, if your body can't eliminate them. If constipation is your problem, see the chapter on constipation in this book.

2. Anemia

Anemia, or a deficiency of hemoglobin in the blood, is one of the major reasons for feeling rundown and tired. It is usually caused by a lack of vital nutrients, which inhibits your body's ability to produce an adequate blood supply. Anemia can also be caused by excessive blood loss. Check with your doctor — a routine blood test will show a low red blood cell and low hemoglobin count.

Symptoms Of Anemia Can Include:

Poor concentration

Thinning hair

Brittle nails

Paleness

Difficulty breathing when climbing stairs

If you suffer from anemia, you need to include iron-rich foods in your diet. Following are common, healthy foods, any of which provide 5 mg. of easily-digestible iron:

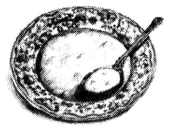

1/2 cup cream of wheat cereal

1/4 block of soya tofu

1/2 cup of cooked soybeans

1/2 cup of raw sunflower seeds

1/4 cup of raw sesame seeds

1 cup of cooked lentils or peas

6 ounces of tuna fish

3 ounces of beef liver

1 1/2 cups of cooked spinach

1 1/2 cups of cooked swiss chard

1/2 cup of dried apricots

3 teaspoons of blackstrap molasses

1 cup of raisins or prunes

In general your diet should include lots of green leafy vegetables, whole grains, and legumes each day.

If diet doesn't alleviate your symptoms, you may suffer from a more specific nutrient deficiency in which case you may need vitamin B-12, B-6 or folic acid. Consult your doctor for help with these supplements.

3. Oxygen Deficiency

Sometimes, when you are feeling tired, even a blood test will not reveal anything wrong with you. It may be that you have an oxygen deficiency. These are some of the symptoms:

Frequent sighing

Feelings of suffocation

Black and blue marks from the slightest bruise

Constant drowsiness and yawning

If you suspect oxygen deficiency, here are three vitamins that may help you get back that get up and go that got up and went:

a) Vitamin C — 500 mg. one pill three times a day with meals.

b) Vitamin E — 400 IU one pill a day.

c) Vitamin B-15 — 50 mg. one pill a day.

4. Low Blood Pressure

Many people are born with low blood pressure. Doctors often feel this is a preferred condition because as people age, blood pressure tends to rise. And high blood pressure is a dangerous condition.

A large percentage of your blood is made up of water. If you have low blood pressure, you need to drink a lot of water to maintain pressure in your bloodstream. People with low blood pressure who do not watch their liquid intake tend to be tired more often, sedentary and listless. Fingertips and toes also can become quite cold because of this condition.

Ask your doctor to take your blood pressure. (There are

also kits available that let you do it yourself.) Normal blood pressure tends to hover around the 120/80 figure. Anything less than 90 for the top figure, and 70 for the bottom figure, is considered low blood pressure.

Blood Pressure And The Heart

One of the more serious problems faced by people with low blood pressure is the strain it puts on the heart. Normal blood pressure helps the heart work at its optimum level. Constant low blood pressure strains the heart by forcing it to work harder to do its job. This can lead to a number of problems.

The Heart Helpers

Vitamin E dilates the coronary blood vessels and enhances cardiac performance. You can get vitamin E naturally, through the food you eat, or in pill form:

a) Vitamin E — 400 IU one pill a day.

b) Cooked whole wheat contains lots of vitamin E and is an excellent food for countering low blood pressure.

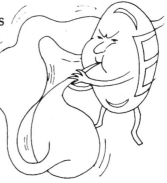

c) Unprocessed cold-pressed vegetable oils such as sunflower oil, sesame oil, and olive oil are excellent sources of natural vitamin E. Eat two-three tablespoons daily in salad dressing or on cooked foods.

Calcium gives tone to the heart muscle and helps to regulate the heartbeat. Here are the best ways to get extra calcium into your system:

a) Calcium Ascorbate which combines 50 mg. calcium and 500 mg. vitamin C. Take one pill, twice a day.

b) Milk products, sesame seeds, most beans, carrots, cabbage, and soya products are rich in calcium.

Blood Pressure And The Adrenal Glands

People with low blood pressure have to be conscious of any sort of adrenal insufficiency. The adrenals are two small glands that sit on top of the kidneys and produce a number of vital hormones, including adrenaline.

Adrenaline constricts blood vessels thereby raising your blood pressure. If the adrenal glands become weakened from stress, too much sugar, or a sedentary lifestyle, your blood pressure will not be elevated when you need it to be. Low blood pressure caused by adrenal insufficiency can make your life miserable. Exercise, even getting out of bed in the morning, could cause dizziness or blackouts.

Pump Them Up

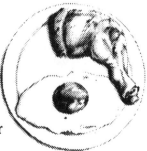

The adrenal glands serve as a storage tank for vitamins B and C. They need protein to function at their maximum. Here's how to keep your adrenal glands in proper working order:

a) Fish, chicken and eggs are the best sources of dietary protein for the adrenals. Choose one serving per day.

b) Licorice root tincture — 20 drops twice daily in water.

c) Vitamin C — 500 mg. one pill twice a day with meals.

5. Enzyme Deficiency

Some people eat all the right foods but still have no energy. Clearly, you cannot get energy from the foods you eat unless your digestive system is working at maximum warp. If you feel that your body is not giving you the energy you expect, it may be that your digestive enzymes, which break down the food you eat, are weak or lacking.

Here are two excellent enzyme supplements that may be helpful. Try them for three months:

a) Bromelain (from pineapple) — 50 mg. one pill twice a day, after meals.

b) Papain (from papaya) — 50 mg. one pill twice a day, after meals.

6. Low Blood Sugar

I have treated thousands of patients with hypoglycemia, more commonly called low blood sugar. Invariably, when I put them on the diet outlined below, they ask me the same question:

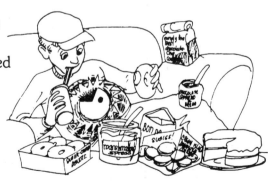

"Why should I eliminate sugar from my diet if my problem is low blood sugar?"

My answer also tends to be the same: "Your body is causing your low blood sugar by reacting to your sugar intake, or rather, over-reacting."

Here's how.

Insulin, which is secreted by the pancreas, works to get sugar from your blood into your body cells where the sugar is then used for energy. The more sugar you eat, the harder your pancreas works to release the insulin needed to get the sugar to your cells.

So far so good. Now we get to the main problem.

Certain sugars, like white sugar, honey, and candy, enter into the bloodstream more rapidly than others, sparking the pancreas to release large amounts of insulin. Sometimes, the pancreas will release more insulin into your bloodstream than is necessary. This is called insulin stress.

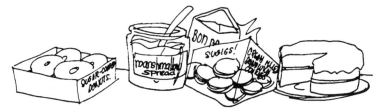

When this occurs, the sugar is being moved out of your blood so quickly that the brain, which needs sugar every minute of every day, starts screaming for more. You begin to experience headaches, dizziness, fainting, and may become confused. Your body craves the sugar that your brain needs to function properly.

So you eat more sugar. And the insulin is released again. It lowers your sugar level, a bit too much. This causes your brain to demand more sugar. And so on and so on...it becomes a vicious circle, with you the loser.

So, the only way to break out of this circle is to find sugars that don't bombard the bloodstream all at once, sugars that enter the bloodstream slowly, allowing the pancreas to release insulin slowly, over a period of time.

The natural sugars found in bread do not enter the blood so quickly. Protein foods like chicken, fish and eggs, as well as beans, peas, and lentils have a sugar-stabilizing effect. Fatty foods, which stay in the stomach longer, prevent sugar from getting into the blood too fast, and are also helpful in stabilizing sugar levels.

The Low-blood-sugar Diet

Using the diet below it is possible to cure, and even prevent a low blood sugar condition. Of course, it is always advisable to take a glucose tolerance test, administered by your doctor, if you feel you have such a condition.

a) Eat three meals per day plus healthy snacks in-between.

b) Do not eat sweets for energy.

c) Eat something from the following list either as a between-meal snack or as a small meal:

Fifteen raw almonds with some raisins. Chew them well.

One small carton of ready-made soya milk.

Whole wheat sandwich or crackers with avocado, peanut butter or tahina.

A handful of any raw nuts or seeds.

One hardboiled egg.

One soyaburger.

Yogurt with fresh fruit.

A bowl of bean soup.

A small piece of fish or chicken.

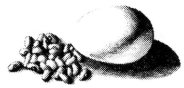

d) Use the following food supplements as well:

Licorice root tincture — 15 drops two to three times a day in any beverage.

Vitamin B-5 (pantothenic acid) — 100 mg. one pill twice a day with meals.

Vitamin C — 500 mg. one pill twice a day with meals.

Spirulina — 350 mg. two tablets three times a day.

All Purpose Anti-fatigue Program

If you are not quite sure why you are fatigued, even after reading this chapter, get a medical check-up. If that still does not work, try my All Purpose Anti-Fatigue Program. Many teens have had amazing success with this program. Try it for three months and see if you don't feel more peppy as well.

1. Eliminate all sweets and junk food.

2. Eat fish, chicken or eggs, daily.

3. Add more raw vegetables like alfalfa sprouts, mung bean sprouts, shredded carrots and romaine lettuce.

4. Include oatmeal, almonds and raisins, egg yolk (don't worry about the cholesterol unless you have a high cholesterol count already), and bean sprouts.

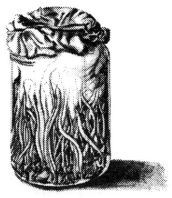

Bean Sprouts

5. Choose one of the following:

a) Bee pollen pills — two pills twice daily with meals.

b) Spirulina pills — 350 mg. two tablets twice daily with meals.

6. Oxygenate your blood:

    a) Exercise daily for at least 15 minutes a day.

    b) Take Vitamin E — 400 IU one pill a day at lunch.

    c) Take Vitamin C — 500 mg. one pill twice a day with meals.

7. Ease the load on your digestive system by:

    a) Following the food combinations suggested in the chapter, What are Healthy Foods?

    b) Taking papaya or pineapple enzymes as discussed in the Enzyme Deficiency section above.

Chapter Ten

Hair Loss

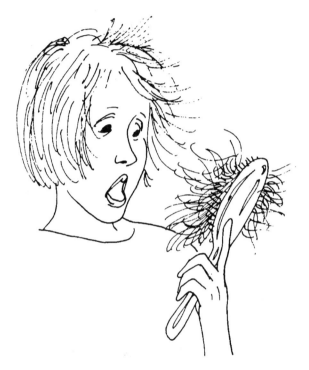

Isaac was a very pleasant 16-year-old. On the phone he had said he was having trouble in school due to some "personal, serious problem I need to speak to you about... privately." His tone was so secretive I was sure he was into drugs.

Isaac walked in, not at all as I imagined, wearing a large Rangers' cap that covered his entire head.

"Nice to meet you," I said. "Tell me what's wrong."

Slowly, Isaac took off his hat. It became immediately clear that he was balding. It was also clear that he was ashamed of his condition.

"All is not lost," I said, looking at his thinning hair. "I've seen less become more."

"Thanks for the encouragement," he said, smiling and quickly replaced his cap.

Basic Causes Of Hair Loss

Almost everyone is upset when they find they are losing hair, but for teenagers it is especially disturbing. Some, like Isaac, try and hide their hair loss. Other boys accept their situation but when they are bombarded with advertisements showing virile young men with a full head of hair, they are left wondering about their own masculinity.

Needless to say, for girls, hair loss, while less common, is just as traumatic. Glistening, vibrant hair is what is expected of a teenage girl. All the ads say so.

Of course, everyone loses some hair every day. If you rub your hair and see some fall out, don't worry. It's natural. If you pull your hair (gently) and a handful comes out, you have a problem.

But don't panic. There are a variety of reasons for balding or hair loss. First, understand the cause of your specific problem, then follow the treatments prescribed. You may be able to treat your hair loss as well as prevent it in the future.

Here are the basic causes of hair loss:

1. Poor Circulation To The Head

Sometimes the blood circulation to the tiny hair follicles of the scalp is cut off. This causes a prolonged absence of precious blood nutrients to the scalp. A scalp deprived of blood becomes tight and thick, leading to the death of hair follicles and the onset of baldness.

The following cause vasoconstriction (closing of blood vessels) and cut off the blood circulation to the hair follicles:

Cigarette smoking
Prolonged stress
High blood pressure
Lack of exercise
Extremely cold temperatures

How To Open Your Blood Vessels

Here are a number of things you can do to open the blood vessels in the scalp:

a) Brewers yeast, high in natural vitamin B-3, better known as Niacin — one tablet twice a day before meals.

b) Vitamin E — 400 IU one tablet twice a day. All natural-source Vitamin E is derived from wheat germ.

Whole wheat cereal provides you with natural Vitamin E.

c) Do shoulder stands. This assures a good blood supply to the head.

d) Lay on a slanted board, head down. This reverses the negative effects of gravity and increases circulation to the scalp.

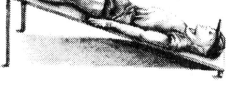

2. Nutritional Deficiencies

The quality of your hair depends a great deal on the foods you eat. Junkfood produces dull, lifeless hair, which is brittle and falls out easily.

Research has shown a positive relationship between hair and B-vitamins. Among the B-vitamins that stand out in their "hair-raising" abilities are biotin, choline, inositol, folic acid and vitamin B-6.

Got a cowlick? Biotin, a B-vitamin, will help tame those wild hairs that just never seem to lie down no matter how much you comb them. Biotin is included among the other B-vitamins in a B-complex supplement.

Adequate protein is also required for the body to build hair, as well as the minerals sulphur and iodine.

Nutritional Treatment

To put life back into your lackluster hair and help encourage growth, you should try the following:

a) B-complex vitamins derived from rice or food-grown-source one pill twice a day.

b) Eggs and beans (in moderation) provide high quality protein plus sulphur, which is important for healthy hair and skin. Be sure to include them in your diet.

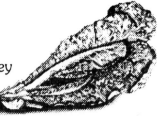

c) Eat green leafy vegetables such as lettuce, cabbage and spinach. They contain large amounts of B-vitamins. The husks of whole wheat and whole brown rice are also an excellent source of B-vitamins.

d) Soya lecithin granules are concentrated sources of B-vitamins. Sprinkle one tablespoon of lecithin granules onto any food, twice daily.

e) Fish provides high quality protein and iodine.

In The Olden Days

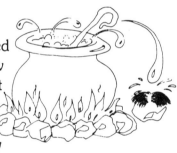

Folk medicines are usually based on trial and error. People didn't know why, but some natural medicines just seemed to work.

Here are a number of foods that seem to promote hair growth by virtue of their rich multi-mineral content. For many people they actually help cure hair loss.

First try any two of the following medicinal foods for about three months. If you don't get the results you want, choose another two, and so on. Trial and error worked in the olden days.

It may work for you too.

a) Apple cider vinegar as a substitute for white vinegar.

b) Oatmeal cereal with one tablespoon added wheat bran.

c) Use blackstrap molasses as a sugar substitute.

d) Bee pollen granules — one teaspoon twice daily, or two

pills twice daily. Bee pollen is a natural food rich in amino-acids, B-vitamins and minerals.

e) Rosemary leaf tea — one teaspoon steeped in one cup of boiled water. Drink warm, one cup, twice a day.

3. Sluggish Thyroid

The thyroid gland controls body metabolism, heart rate and body temperature. A weakened thyroid can cause:

Coarse, brittle or dry hair

Hair that falls out easily when combed

Thinning eyebrows

If you suspect your thyroid is not doing its job — ask your physician to check it out through a routine blood test.

Feed Your Thyroid Right

Nutrition alone can do much to restore a weak thyroid gland and often produces remarkable recovery of hair. The following foods are helpful for this purpose:

a) Ocean fish, fresh or frozen.

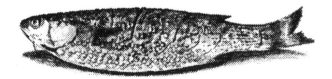

b) Seaweed, such as kombu, which may be purchased from health food stores. Add one piece daily to any soup.

c) Onions and egg yolks are high in natural iodine which is necessary for the thyroid to produce its hormones.

4. Fever/Shock

Certain circumstances, such as fever or sudden emotional shock, may cause a dramatic loss of hair.

Hair lost due to fever grows back on its own, in a short time, after the fever has passed.

Hair loss due to sudden emotional shock is not so easily remedied. The shock and emotional issues need to be dealt with.

5. Improper Hair Care

What you do to your hair with dyes, harsh shampoos and hot air dryers, affects the way it looks and how long it lasts.

Be Kind To Your Hair

a) Switch to natural non-synthetic hair color to avoid the damaging effects of synthetic dyes.

b) Use natural shampoos, instead of harsh shampoos, preferably one containing biotin, a B-vitamin.

c) Make your own shampoo. Every day, 10 minutes before showering, rub one or two egg yolks into your scalp and hair. Let the mixture sit for 10 minutes and then wash it off. You will be immediately impressed with the results.

d) Avoid hot air dryers. They can cause a lot of damage to your hair.

Homemade Hair Growth Tonic

Many teens have been pleased with the results of this powerful hair tonic.

Ingredients:

- 40 grams each of dried herbs: rosemary, horsetail, sage and nettles

- 2 1/2 cups of vodka (50 proof). No tasting! Remember this is to get your hair to grow, not stand on its end.

Steps:

1. Place all ingredients into a sealed glass container. Put in a dark place for two weeks.

2. Shake twice daily.

3. After two weeks strain off all liquid and throw away the herbs.

4. Vigorously massage entire scalp with tonic before going to sleep. Leave tonic on scalp overnight and wash off in the morning.

5. Use tonic for at least one month to give it a chance to work.

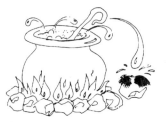

Chapter Eleven
Brainpower

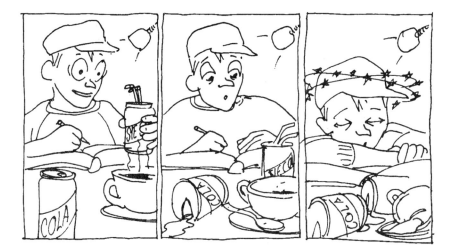

Mental Performance
Memory Enhancement

Joshua is a genius. His I.Q. is somewhere in the 160s.

But he complains that he can't concentrate. He is absent-minded, and for all his potential brilliance, he claims to have a very poor short-term memory.

What's wrong?

Lots of people have high potential. They *could* be great or strong or wealthy. But potential just means you can do it. Performance, on the other hand, means you *are* doing it. To be successful you have to utilize your potential.

And that depends on various factors, particularly the food you put into your body. Nutrition not only affects your physical performance, but also has a profound effect on your mental performance.

Joshua's High

For energy, Joshua would drink three or four cups of coffee by lunch time. He claimed it gave him just the right "high" to be able to get through his first three periods, including French. For lunch Joshua gulped down his meal with a cola chaser, sometimes two.

By early afternoon his system — which had become used to this caffeine regimen — neutralized all the caffeine he had been pumping into it...and Joshua came crashing down. He became tired, unable to concentrate, irritable and annoyed with everyone and everything.

There's no question that caffeine gives you that extra little boost some of us may need in the morning, or the middle of the day. Caffeine speeds up the neurotransmitters of the brain so you can shake off your grogginess and take that test feeling refreshed. It lets you get that extra hour of study late at night when the phone has stopped ringing and everyone else is in bed. However, when its effects wear off, watch out! The results can be disastrous.

Why? Because caffeine has no nutritional signifi- cance. It's a drug which lasts for a short time and then...crash!

Brain Minerals

The real nutritional contributions to mind performance come from foods high in the "brain minerals" magnesium and manganese.

Foods High in Magnesium

Egg yolk (best soft boiled)

Yellow cornmeal cereal

Whole-grain cooked cereals (whole wheat, whole rice)

Dried prunes and figs

Foods High in Manganese:

Walnuts

Pecans

Peas and lentils

The brain also requires phosphorous, another mineral, which is abundant in protein foods and therefore supplements are not necessary. Protein foods most recommended for brainpower are fish and egg yolks.

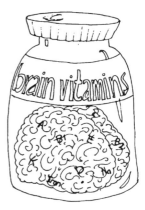

Brain Vitamins

The B-vitamins are also important for mental performance, especially choline and inositol which occur naturally in a fat called lecithin. Foods high in lecithin include egg yolk, avocado and soybeans.

It is best to buy a natural B-complex supplement from a rice-source. (Rice polishings, or skins, contain the vitamins discarded in the production of white rice.)

Here's what I recommend. Choose only one form of lecithin.

1. Lecithin granules — one tablespoon eaten twice a day. (sprinkled on top of any food, has a nutty flavor).
2. Lecithin capsules — 1200 mg. twice a day with meals.
3. B-complex (rice-source) — one tablet a day with meals.

Brain Cocktails - L'chaim!

Choose one of the following "cocktails" each day. Joshua began noticing an improvement in his mental abilities soon after taking these regularly.

1. One glass of canned pineapple juice with one tablespoon of rice polishings.
2. One glass of goat's milk.
3. Fish soup as an afternoon meal with plenty of cooked and raw vegetables.

Herbal Medicine

Various herbal potions have been used throughout history to boost brainpower. I have had the most success with the following:

1. Gotu Kola (Centella Asiatica).This amazing herb has been used for thousands of years in the Orient. It promotes mental clarity and long life. It is a natural stimulant of the central nervous system and has been employed by herbalists as an anti-depressant and anti-fatigue remedy. It is available in both tea form and tincture. The most effective way to take this remedy is to purchase the tincture and add 15 drops to a glass of water several times a day.

2. Ginko Bilboa. Your brain needs a constant supply of oxygen which it receives from the blood. The more oxygen-rich your blood becomes, the better your brain will operate. This herb is especially effective in improving cerebral blood circulation and consequently oxygenation. Take one capsule twice daily with water.

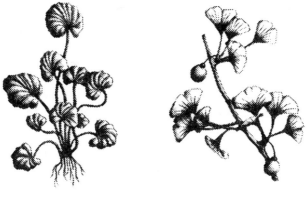

Gotu Kola   *Ginko Bilboa*

Memory Enhancement

Miriam complained of absentmindedness and poor memory. She thought she was getting Alzheimers disease. I explained to her that very few people contract this disease at 14 years of age.

I sat with her for over an hour outlining a specific program of nutrition and natural ingredients that I felt would be best suited for her. I filled three pages with diagrams and notes for her to refer to.

At the end of our session, she thanked me and left my office. When I returned to my chair I noticed she had left the sheets on my desk.

Why are some people so forgetful?

Remember Amino Acids

The brain requires certain minerals to function properly.

Magnesium, manganese and phosphorous are important. Proteins, which are composed of some 26 individual amino acid building blocks, provide substance for brain fuel.

High school students can assure themselves of adequate protein intake by including a general amino acid formula, in pill form, in their daily diet. Use amino acid pills from either a soy or egg source. (Follow instructions on the bottle.)

These days, health professionals have devoted a lot of time and interest to one amino acid in particular: L-Glutamine. Among the 26 amino acids, this one stands out for its ability to enhance mental performance.

L-Glutamine — 500 mg. once a day.

Breathing and Exercise

The basic elements that the brain needs every minute of every day are oxygen and sugar. Depriving a newborn baby of oxygen for a few minutes can result in permanent brain damage.

The oxygen needed by the brain is diffused through the blood. But adequate oxygen in the blood depends on breathing which, in turn, is dependent on how much you exercise.

If your brain has insufficient oxygen, there is something you can do. Exercise to the point of increased breathing rate. Even a few minutes of this helps, if performed daily, to build up adequate oxygen reserves for your brain.

Another way to increase circulation to the brain is to lay on an inverted exercise board with your head in a downward position and the feet elevated approximately 18 inches off the floor:

Relaxing in this position brings needed blood to the brain. (This method should not be used by anyone with high blood pressure.)

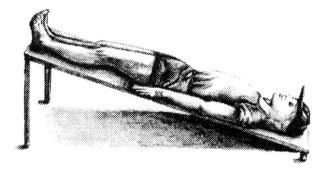

The Lazy Way Out

Remember Joshua? He couldn't understand the benefits of exercise.

"Why get all sweaty?" he said. "Let the fat kids exercise. I'm perfectly happy with my body."

"But is your body happy with you?" I asked. "Are you treating it the way you should? You complain about being tired and upset in the afternoons. Maybe your body needs an oxygen pick-me-up, rather than a caffeine fix, for a change. Get some exercise!"

"Just give me some pills or something. Let me worry about my body," came the swift reply.

For those of you who feel the same way, here are some excellent supplements you can take to help oxygenate your blood:

1. Coenzyme Q — 50 mg. per day increases brain oxygen.

2. Vitamin E — 400 IU once a day.

Researchers have proven the positive effects of B-vitamins

on memory. Vitamin B-6 (pyridoxine), and Vitamin B-5 (pantothenic acid) increase the quantity of neurotransmitters in the brain. Vitamin B-3 (niacin) improves circulation of blood to the brain. A good B-complex supplement from food-grown or rice source should include all of these. Take one tablet, twice daily. But remember, these vitamins don't make you smarter — just quicker.

The Need for Sugar

The other vital element necessary for your brain to function at its top capacity is sugar. Without the correct sugar levels your brain becomes fatigued. If the levels of sugar are too low you begin to suffer the symptoms of hypoglycemia (low blood sugar) which include:

> Sudden forgetfulness
> Inability to concentrate
> Physical fatigue
> Depression
> Lack of motivation

I cannot overemphasize the effects low blood sugar has on memory and brain performance. For a more detailed look on how eating more sweets actually gives you low blood sugar and what happens to your body, take a good look at the chapter dealing with fatigue.

Brewers Yeast

Last but not least there is an element in brewers yeast and certain foods such as sardines and salmon called nutritional RNA (ribonucleic acid). Brewers yeast is a natural source of all the B-vitamins and has a high content of RNA making it a natural memory booster.

Brewers yeast pills — twice a day.

Unfortunately, maybe 30 percent of my clients are allergic to yeast products. If you suspect that you have an allergy to yeast products, do not take this supplement.

Chapter Twelve

Recipes

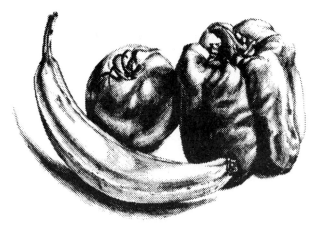

All the ingredients you need for these recipes can be purchased at your local healthfood store, and many of them are even available at the supermarket.

Be sure to buy only whole grains, not processed grains or cereals, to get the most nutritional value out of your food.

GRAINS

Brown Rice

   1 cup brown rice
   3 cups water

1. Soak the rice overnight in water (enough to cover).

2. In the morning, drain off water and toss.

3. Add three cups fresh water.

4. Bring to a boil and lower the flame.

5. Add a pinch of salt and simmer, covered, for 40 minutes.

Millet

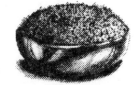

1 cup millet
3 cups water

1. Soak the millet overnight in water (enough to cover).

2. In the morning, drain off water and toss.

3. Add three cups of fresh water

4. Bring to a boil and lower flame.

5. Add a pinch of salt and simmer, covered, for 30 minutes.

Bulgur Wheat

1 cup bulgur wheat
3 cups water

1. Soak the wheat overnight in water (enough to cover).

2. In the morning, drain off the water and toss.

3. Add three cups fresh water

4. Bring to a boil and lower the flame.

5. Add a pinch of salt and simmer, covered, for 40 minutes.

Buckwheat Cereal (Kasha)

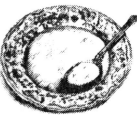

1 cup buckwheat groats
2-1/2 cups water

1. Soak buckwheat in water overnight.

2. In morning, bring to a boil, lower flame and simmer, covered, for 10 minutes.

Cornmeal·Cereal

1 cup yellow cornmeal
4 cups water

1. Boil the water and lower flame.
2. Add the cornmeal and simmer for 20 minutes, stirring constantly to avoid lumps.

BREAD

Homemade Whole Wheat Bread

Makes two loaves

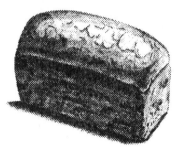

Step One:
2 cups whole wheat flour
2 packages active dry yeast
1 tablespoon molasses
1 teaspoon salt
2 cups warm water

Step Two:
2-1/2 cups whole wheat flour
2 tablespoons lecithin

1. Mix ingredients in Step One together and allow to stand for 10 minutes.
2. Beat the mixture by hand or with an electric mixer.
3. Cover and allow to stand for 15 minutes.
4. Add ingredients from Step Two.
5. Knead the dough well. Make sure it doesn't stick, adding more flour if necessary.

6. Shape into two good-sized loaves. Raise in pans until the loaves double in size.

7. Bake for 45 minutes at 350°.

8. Allow to cool completely before eating.

SOUPS

Miso Soup

4 cups of water
6 teaspoons Miso paste
1 tablespoon sesame oil
2 onions

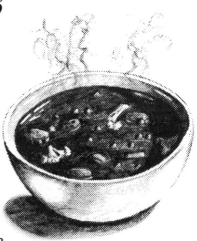

1. Saute the onions in oil.

2. Place the sauted onions and four cups of water in a pot.

3. Bring to a boil and lower flame.

4. Mix one cup of the boiled water and Miso paste together.

5. Put the Miso water back in to the main pot and simmer for eight minutes. Do not let the soup boil.

Vegetable Soup

3 quarts of water
1 quart tomatoes, chopped
1 cup brown rice, uncooked
1 cup green beans
2 stalks celery, chopped
2 cups squash, winter (cubed)
1 tablespoon onion powder

1. Bring water to a boil.
2. Add all ingredients and return to a boil.
3. Lower flame and simmer, covered, for one hour.
4. Green beans may be added during the last half hour of cooking to retain their color.
5. Add one tablespoon of cold-pressed oil and a handful of chopped parsley before serving.

Pea Soup

1 cup dry split peas
2 carrots, diced
1 onion, chopped
2 celery stalks, chopped
1 teaspoon vegetable salt
1 clove garlic
2 tablespoons olive oil

1. Cover the dried peas with water and soak overnight.
2. In the morning, drain and toss the water.
3. Add five cups of fresh water.
4. Add all the vegetables, cover the pot and cook until the peas are mushy (stirring often to prevent clumps).
5. When soup is ready, add two tablespoons olive oil.
6. Run the whole mixture through a blender for a smoother product.

Tomato Soup With Onions

 6 tomatoes
 3 onions
 1/2 cup parsley, chopped

1. Steam the vegetables for about 10 minutes.
2. Place the steamed vegetables into a pot with three cups of water and simmer on low heat for another eight minutes (do not boil).
3. Add vegetable seasoning, to taste.

High Potassium Vegetable Broth

 2 cups potatoes (with skins), sliced
 2 cups carrots, thinly sliced
 2 cups turnips, thinly sliced
 1 onion, sliced
 Outside leaves of cabbage
 Stalks of asparagus

1. Wash vegetables and discard wilted parts.
2. Slice and put into large saucepan.
3. Cover with water and bring to boil.
4. Reduce heat and let simmer, covered, for two hours.
5. Strain, salt to taste and garnish with chopped fresh parsley.
6. This broth may also be used as a base for other soups.

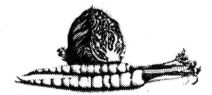

Lima Bean Soup

1 pound lima beans, dry
3 quarts water
4 cups celery, chopped
1 cup tomatoes
1/2 cup onion, chopped, or
    1 tablespoon onion powder
1-1/2 teaspoon salt, to taste

1. Soak beans and celery in water for 4-5 hours.

2. Bring to a boil and add tomatoes, onion and salt.

3. Cook until tender.

4. Add two tablespoons olive oil.

5. Dilute with water if desired.

Lentil Soup

1 cup green lentils
1 medium onion
1 can tomato juice
1/2 clove garlic
1 carrot
2 celery stalks
1 green pepper
1 teaspoon salt

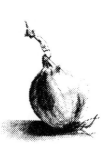

1. Soak the lentils in water overnight.

2. In the morning, drain off the water and toss.

3. Chop all the vegetables and put into a pot with lentils.

4. Cover with several inches of water and cook on a low flame, covered, for 3-4 hours.

5. Add the tomato juice at the end of the cooking time.

SALADS, DRESSINGS & SPREADS

Grow Your Own Sprouts

Sprouts are probably the most basic and vital food you can eat in our polluted world. It's fun and easy to grow your own.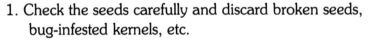

All you need are good quality seeds, a large wide-mouth glass jar, and a piece of wire mesh, cheesecloth or a special sprouting lid.

1. Check the seeds carefully and discard broken seeds, bug-infested kernels, etc.

2. Clean the seeds by rinsing them several times with water.

3. Soak most seeds in a dark place for 12 hours (summer) or 15 hours (winter). Smaller seeds like alfalfa require only 8-12 hours.

4. Drain off all water through the wire or cheesecloth. Cover the seeds with water again and rinse thoroughly. Be sure to drain off all excess water.

5. Place the sprout jar in an upside-down position, tilted so that excess water can drain off during the day. Cover the jar with a towel.

6. Rinse and drain the sprouts twice daily until they are ready.

7. Knowing when the sprouts are ready can be a bit tricky. They are usually ready when the sprout is at least twice the length of the seed. You can consult a sprouting manual for exact descriptions.

8. Enjoy your sprouts plain, on salads, in sandwiches, or any way you can think of.

Vegetable Salad

Mix a variety of raw vegetables together into a tasty salad. Try all kinds of mixtures.

Tahina Dressing

1. Dilute tahina with water until it has the consistency of a pourable sauce, or dressing.
2. Add a little tamari (soya) sauce or lemon for flavor.

COOKED VEGETABLES

Three Methods

To ensure the highest vitamin retention from your produce, buy fresh vegetables (frozen if you must), wash them immediately, dry and refrigerate.

Cutting the vegetables into shreds or small pieces will reduce the cooking time needed to steam or stir-fry them. Choose one of the following cooking techniques.

1. Steamed Vegetables - the healthiest

1. Put prepared vegetables into a steamer basket that inserts in any pan.
2. Put about one cup water into the bottom of the pan and bring to a boil.
3. Insert the steamer basket, lower the flame and cover the pan.

4. Cook the vegetables just slightly past the time of their deepest color. Carrots turn bright orange, broccoli turns deep green, etc. The whole process takes anywhere from 5-15 minutes depending on how starchy the vegetable and the size of the pieces.

2. Baked Vegetables

Vegetables can be placed directly in the oven or wrapped in parchment paper and baked.

Potatoes should always be baked. Whole beets and other strong root vegetables are surprisingly tasty when prepared this way.

3. Stir-fried Vegetables - the natural alternative for you fried-food addicts.

Normally, frying foods requires heating the oil to an extreme temperature which makes the oil harder to digest. Stir-fry, my variation on the classic Oriental method of cooking, requires less heat but more care.

1. Put enough water in a frying pan or wok to just cover the bottom of the pan. Heat the water to boiling.

2. Add a small amount of oil on top of the boiling water and heat.

3. Add the cut vegetables to the pan and stir constantly the entire cooking time until the vegetables are full-colored and just tender. The length of cooking time will depend on which vegetables you use.

Fermented Vegetables

These are available as sauerkraut or sour pickles, ready-made, from the healthfood store. Be sure to buy only a brand that does not use vinegar.

Baked Red Potatoes With Olive Oil And Cayenne Pepper

1. Bake the potatoes, whole, in the oven.

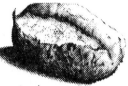

2. Before eating, open them up and add olive oil and cayenne pepper. (Do not cook the oil or cayenne pepper.)

MAIN DISHES

Spaghetti With Soy Pieces And Tomato Sauce

1. Prepare whole wheat spaghetti according to directions on package.
2. Purchase any tomato sauce, without preservatives, or ready-made natural spaghetti sauce.
3. Buy dry soy pieces from healthfood store and boil them in water for 10 minutes.
4. Heat the tomato sauce with some water and add one tablespoon tamari (soya) sauce.
5. Serve the spaghetti together with soy pieces and the sauce.

Tempe/Tofu

You can purchase tempe and/or tofu ready-made from the health food store.

1. Cook the tempe following instructions on the package.
2. Saute pieces of tofu in sesame oil.
3. Mix the tofu and tempe together for a "meaty" meatless meal.
4. Garnish with a few sprigs of parsley.

Tofu With Tamari

Buy tofu, ready-made, from the healthfood store or oriental food store. Many supermarkets also carry this soy food.

1. Cut the tofu into small pieces.
2. Saute the cubes in a pan with sesame oil and tamari (soya sauce).
3. Serve them with anything as a meat, cheese or egg substitute.

Beans

Cook beans in either a pressure cooker or stainless steel or pyrex pot.

1. Soak 2-1/2 cups of beans in water overnight.
2. In the morning, throw away the water and rinse beans.
3. Place the beans in a pot with 3-1/2 cups water and 1/2 teaspoon salt.
4. Bring the water to a boil, lower the flame and cook beans on a low flame, covered, until they are tender and ready to eat (1-2 hours).

Azuki Beans

1. Soak 2-1/2 cups azuki beans in water overnight.
2. In the morning, throw away the water and rinse the beans.
3. Place beans in a pot with 3-1/2 cups of water and 1/2 teaspoon salt.
4. Bring water to a boil, lower the flame and cook the beans, partially covered, until they are tender and ready to eat (1-2 hours).

Baked White Fish

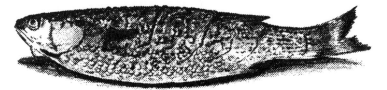

(use fresh or frozen white fish — no carp or fatty type)
1. Oil a broiling rack and preheat broiler.
2. Baste the fish with tomato sauce, lemon juice, or wine.
3. Cook the fish for 10 minutes, turning it only once.

Baked Poultry

Cooking poultry at high (350° +) temperatures makes it difficult to digest. It is best to use high temperatures for only a short time or use low (200°) temperatures for a long period of time.

1. Place a whole chicken or turkey in a large pot with tomato sauce and onions.

2. Cook uncovered for 20 minutes at 350°.

3. Cover pot and reduce heat to 200°.

4. Continue cooking until the meat is tender. About 2-1/2 hours for a small chicken and 3-1/2 hours for a small turkey.

Any of the following methods can be used to cook eggs to their optimum state of solid white and runny yolks.

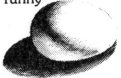

Soft Boiled Eggs

Put the whole egg, in shell, into boiling water and simmer for 3-5 minutes.

Steamed Eggs

Put the eggs in a steamer basket, just like vegetables and steam them until done.

Poached Eggs

1. Place water in a shallow pan and bring to a boil.

2. Turn off the fire.

3. Crack an egg into a dish and gently slide the egg into the water.

4. Cover the pan and let stand for 15 minutes or until the egg whites are solid.

Lentil Casserole

1-1/2 cups dry lentils
1/2 cup whole wheat bread crumbs
1 cup tomatoes, mashed
1 onion, finely chopped
1 clove garlic, diced
1/2 cup celery, chopped

1. Soak the lentils overnight in water.
2. In the morning, drain water and toss.
3. Add three cups of fresh water and bring to a boil.
4. Lower the flame and simmer at least one hour until the lentils are tender and soft.
5. Combine all the above ingredients and form into a loaf.
6. Bake in an oiled baking dish for one hour at 350°.

Broccoli With Beans and Spaghetti

1/2 pound northern dry beans
1/2 pound buckwheat or soy spaghetti
2 pounds broccoli
1 large onion, sliced
1 large tomato, chopped
Salt, to taste

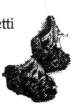

1. Soak and cook beans until tender in 1-1/2 quarts of water with onion and tomato.
2. Cook chopped broccoli in salted water almost until tender.
3. Add the spaghetti (broken into pieces) to the broccoli and water. Let cook, stirring occasionally until both are tender.
4. Add cooked beans, salt to taste and a little oil. Heat to blend flavors and serve.

Garbanzo Croquettes

    1-1/2 cups cooked garbanzo beans (coarsely blended)
    2-1/2 cups steamed brown rice
    2 slices bread, crumbled and soaked in 1/4 cup
      garbanzo broth
    2 tablespoons peanut or nut butter
    1/2 cup pecans, finely chopped
    2 tablespoons onion or 1 tablespoon onion powder
    2 tablespoons tamari (soya) sauce
    2 tablespoons oil
    1/2 teaspoon vegetable salt
    Bread crumbs to make desired consistency

1. Mix all ingredients well with hands and form into croquettes or patties.

2. Roll in bread crumbs and sprinkle with oil.

3. Bake at 375° for 45 minutes.

Tofu And Rice Croquettes

    4 cups steamed brown rice
    4 cups tofu
    1/2 cup peanut butter
    2 teaspoons salt
    2 tablespoons oil
    1 tablespoon onion powder
    3 tablespoons tamari (soya) sauce
    1 cup chopped parsley

1. Mix together in given order.

2. Add seasonings, to taste.

3. Form into croquettes or patties and sprinkle with paprika.
4. Bake at 350°-375°, turning to brown on all sides.

SWEETS

Coconut Cashew Bars

1 cup honey or date sugar
1/2 cup oil + 1 teaspoon lecithin
2 tablespoons lemon juice
1/2 cup soy flour
2 cups quick oats
1 cup shredded coconut
1 cup ground cashews
1/4 cup water (more if date sugar is used)
1/2 teaspoon vanilla
1/2 teaspoon salt
1/2 cup chopped pecans or almonds (optional)

1. Combine all ingredients.
2. Mix and press 1/4" thick on an oiled cookie sheet.
3. Bake about at 350° for about 20 minutes.
4. Cut into squares while still hot.

Easy Cooked Granola

9 cups raw oats
2 cups soy flour
1 cup whole wheat flour
1/2 cup coconut, shredded

3/4 cup date sugar or honey
1/2 cup oil mixed with
1 cup boiling water
2 teaspoons salt
1 teaspoon vanilla

1. Blend together liquid ingredients.

2. Stir into dry ingredients.

3. Crumble and bake on cookie sheet.

4. Start at 350° for 15 minutes, then lower to 200° and bake until dry and golden brown. Stir occasionally.

5. Store in covered jars. Keeps well.

Chapter Thirteen

Other Problems/Other Remedies

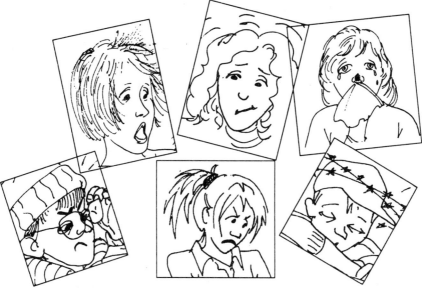

Following are home remedies for a variety of problems, not dealt with in this book. Give them a try, they can be very effective. As always, if the condition persists, or gets worse, you should consult with a natural health practitioner or your doctor.

Acid Feeling in Stomach

a) One tablespoon aloe vera juice in water or herb tea. Drink twice a day.

b) Herb tea — chamomile and mint.

Amoeba (diagnosed by doctor)

a) Acidophilus capsules — take two twice a day, in the early morning and before bed.

b) Garlic capsules — take two three times a day.

Bad Breath

a) Chew on a sprig of parsley (natural chlorophyll) often.

b) Chew on a dried clove, anytime.

Black And Blue Marks (bruise easily)

a) Vitamin C — 500 mg. with bioflavonoids, one pill three times a day.

b) Vitamin E — 400 IU once a day.

Bladder Or Urinary Tract Infection

a) Cranberry juice — drink one cup three times a day.

b) Echinacea capsules — two capsules twice a day.

c) Apple cider vinegar — one teaspoon in water three times a day.

Broken Bones (to speed healing)

a) Herbal tea — one teaspoon each of nettles and horsetail herb. Drink one cup three times a day.

b) Cabbage and carrot juice 50/50 — drink one cup twice a day.

Cold Hands And Feet

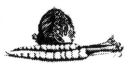

a) 1/4 teaspoon of cayenne pepper (capsicum) in a glass of water. Drink several times a day.

b) Tea — 1/4 teaspoon of cinnamon and 1/8 teaspoon of ginger powder in boiled water. Drink several cups a day.

Dandruff

a) Wash hair with mixture of one tablespoon apple cider vinegar to one cup water.

b) Use a natural shampoo containing rosemary.

Diarrhea

a) Acidophilus — two capsules three times a day.

b) Garlic — two capsules three times a day.

c) Herb tea — one tablespoon of thyme, one teaspoon of mint and 1/8 teaspoon of cinnamon powder in one cup boiled water. Drink freely until the diarrhea stops.

Dry Skin Or Eyes

a) Brewers yeast — one pill three times a day before meals.

b) Beta carotene — 10,000 IU one tablet a day.

Dysentery

a) TREATMENT
Charcoal tablets — two tablets, twice a day.

b) PREVENTION
Acidophilus — two capsules three times a day.
Garlic — two capsules three times a day.

Teen Health • The Natural Way

Ear Infections

a) Garlic oil — squeeze three drops from capsule in ear at night before sleeping.

b) Vitamin C — 1000 mg. twice a day.

c) Echinacea — two capsules twice a day with water.

Eyes Are Red
(many tiny blood vessels in white of eye)

a) Vitamin C — 1000 mg. twice a day.

b) Eat only fruit and vegetables for 24 hours.

c) Beta carotene — 10,000 IU one capsule twice a day.

Eyes Are Tired

Eyebright herb tea — drink one cup, three times daily sweetened with honey.

Gas And Bloating

Tea — one teasoon each of anise, rosemary and mint.

Gums That Bleed Easily

a) Vitamin C — 500 mg. with bioflavanoids, one pill three times a day.

b) Rinse your mouth with baking soda and salt after each brushing. Dissolve one teaspoon baking soda and 1/2 teaspoon salt in 1/2 cup of warm water.

Hives

a) Calcium ascorbate — one pill containing calcium and 500 mg. vitamin C, three times a day.

b) Licorice root tincture — 20 drops twice a day.

Hot Weather Blues
(can't take the summer heat)

a) Apple cider vinegar — one teaspoon in cup of water, twice a day.

b) Carrot-celery juice 50/50 — drink one cup twice a day.

Insomnia

a) Sleepy tea — one teaspoon each of passiflora and camomile in boiling water.

b) Tincture of skullcap — 25 drops in water or herb tea, before bed.

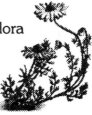

Camomile

Passiflora

Laryngitis

a) Salt water gargle — one teaspoon of seasalt in one cup of warm water — gargle and spit it out.

b) Licorice root tincture (gives strength to the voice) — 25 drops in 1/4 cup of water. Gargle and swallow.

Mosquito Bites (prevention)

a) Apple cider vinegar — one teaspoon in glass of water before bed.

b) Apple cider vinegar — dab onto exposed skin.

Muscle Cramps
(as soon as you feel a cramp coming on)

a) Calcium (500 mg.)-magnesium (250 mg.) tablet — chew on one tablet every 10 minutes, up to four tablets.

b) Cramp bark tincture — 30 drops every 10 minutes, up to three doses.

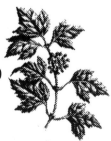

Cramp bark

Nails Cracking/Splitting Or White Spots On Nails

a) Zinc Gluconate — 15 mg. one tablet a day.

b) Calcium Lactate — 500 mg. one tablet a day.

c) Horsetail herb — one tablet a day.

Nausea

a) Ginger root powder — one capsule with one cup strong mint tea.

b) Vitamin B-6 — 50 mg. one pill a day.

Nosebleeds

a) Shepherd's purse herb tea — one teaspoon per cup of boiled water. Drink one cup, twice a day.

b) Rutin — one pill twice a day.

Shoulder Pain

a) Evening primrose oil — two capsules twice a day with meals.

b) Bromelain — 100 mg. three times a day between meals, for three days.

Taste Loss

Zinc gluconate lozenges — suck on one lozenge twice a day.

Tongue (burning feeling)

Vitamin B-complex from rice source — one pill twice a day.

Travel Or Motion Sickness

a) Vitamin B-6 — 50 mg. one tablet twice a day on day of travel.

b) Chew on mint chewing gum.

Warts

a) Vitamin A — 10,000 IU one capsule a day.

b) Castor oil — rub it into the wart twice a day.

Worms/Parasites

Take the following regimen (all three) for 10 days:

a) Acidophilus — two capsules three times a day.

b) Garlic capsules — two capsules three times a day.

c) Shelled pumpkin seeds — eat two tablespoons a day.

About The Author

Yaakov Berman's unique approach to Natural Medicine is due, in large measure, to his own battle with the teenage ailments included in this book. When young people come to him to seek advice, he knows how they feel and what they are going through because he's been there.

Mr. Berman suffered from a debilitating skin disease for over five years and because of this illness was forced to give up a promising career in computer technology. Instead, he took up the study of Nutrition and Natural Medicine, in part to heal his chronic illness. Ultimately, he earned an M.S. in Nutrition and an M.A. in Health Education.

After studying with some of the leading naturopathic physicians and chiropractors in the United States, he was able to overcome his skin disease and from that time on has dedicated his life to the study and teaching of nutrition and health principles, many of which date back in history to the the times of Hippocrates, Galen and the 11th-century genius Rabbi Moses ben Maimon (Maimonides).

In 1974 Yaakov Berman studied with Dr. Bernard Jenson, considered the foremost American authority on iridology (diagnosis of illness via the iris of the eye). Since then, Mr. Berman has pioneered new applications for iridology in conjuction with natural medicine. To this end, he has established a two-year educational program for professionals at the Brui-Teva School, in Tel Aviv, Israel.

Mr. Berman has authored two books, both of which have been translated into Hebrew: *Nutrition and Natural Medicine for Digestive Disease*, 1990, and *Physiologic Approach to Natural*

Medicine, 1994.

He maintains an active practice in Tel Aviv. In addition, he is the nutrition consultant for the Machon Assia Health Center in Jerusalem. Mr. Berman currently lives in Jerusalem with his wife and six children.

Glossary

acidophilus

The healthy bacteria in the intestinal tract.

acupuncture

The practice of placing needles at specific points on the body to help cure disease or relieve pain. Practiced by an acupuncturist.

additives

Substances, usually preservatives, that are added to our food and change its chemical makeup.

adrenal glands

Two small glands that sit on top of the kidneys and produce a number of vital hormones, including adrenaline.

aloe vera

A plant used in the production of cosmetics and skin creams. Repairs damaged skin.

Alzheimers disease

A disease of the central nervous system characterized by premature mental deterioration.

amphetamines

A drug that stimulates the central nervous system.
Frequently used — and abused — as an appetite
suppressant.

anorexia

A serious eating disorder, most commonly found
in young women.

antibodies

Proteins produced by the body's immune system
against foreign bacteria.

bioflavonoids

Part of a vitamin C-complex.

blood pressure

The pressure exerted by the blood on the walls of the
blood vessels, especially the arteries.

blood sugar

Sugar in the form of glucose present in the blood.

bread sugars

Sugars found naturally in bread.

brewers yeast

A source of B-complex vitamins.

bromelain
Enzyme from pineapple.

caffeine
A stimulant found in coffee, tea and kola nuts.

carbohydrates
Found in plants, it includes all sugars, starches and cellulose and is a basic source of human energy.

cardiac
Of or relating to the heart.

cholesterol
A fatty substance produced by the liver that is also found concentrated in various foods.

coenzyme
An enzyme activator.

cold pressed oil
Natural, unprocessed oil that has not been subjected to the usual refining process.

colon
Large intestine, bowel.

cowlick
A lock or tuft of hair growing in a different direction from the rest of the hair.

dysentery

A disease characterized by severe diarrhea.

echinacea

An herb that stimulates the immune function and also
has anti-inflammatory properties.

enzymes

Complex proteins produced by living cells that cause
specific biochemical reactions.

fiber

The indigestible portion of the food you eat.

flora

Bacterial life forms.

fungus

Plant-like organisms that feed on organic matter.

glucose tolerance test

A test to determine the levels of sugar in the blood.

hair follicles

Narrow tubes in the skin, through which hairs grow.

hemoglobin

The iron-containing pigment of the red blood cells.

histamine
> A substance produced by the body during an allergic reaction.

husk
> The shell or outer covering.

hypoglycemia
> Low blood sugar.

immune system
> The body's defense system against sickness.

insulin
> A pancreatic hormone which takes sugar out of the blood and brings it into the cells so it can be used for energy.

IU — International Unit.
> A unit of measurement.

l'chaim
> "To life" in Hebrew. A toast.

lymph
> A circulating body fluid that transports antibodies throughout the body.

metabolism

The transformation in the body of the chemical energy
of foods to mechanical energy or heat.

MSG

Monosodium Glutamate, a salt, flavor enhancer. Often
used in Chinese cooking and processed foods.

Mt. Vesuvius

A volcano that exploded suddenly and violently.

neurotransmitter

A chemical agent that transmits nerve impulses to the
brain.

oxygenation

To supply or combine with oxygen.

pancreas

The gland that produces digestive enzymes which
act in the small intestine to digest protein,
carbohydrate, and fat.

peristaltic wave

Successive waves of continuous contraction along
walls of intestines forcing contents onward.

PMS

Premenstrual Syndrome. A variety of symptoms from which young women may suffer before their menstrual flow.

RDA

Recommended Dietary Allowance as determined by the Food and Nutrition Board of the National Academy of Sciences, National Research Council.

ribonucleic acid

RNA, a protein naturally occurring in various foods.

rutin

A bioflavonoid, part of C-vitamin complex.

sebaceous glands

Glands under the surface of the skin that secrete sebum (oil).

spirulina

A plant protein, from algae.

tahina

Sesame seeds ground into an edible paste.

Tai Chi

Ancient Chinese system of meditative movements practiced as a system of exercises.

tamari

Fermented soy sauce.

tempe

Fermented/cultured soybeans.

tincture

Concentrated solution of plant essence in an alcohol base.

tofu

Soybean curd.

toxic

Poisonous.

vasoconstriction

Constriction, or closure, of the blood vessels.

vasodilation

Dilation, or opening, of the blood vessels.

yoga

System of exercises for attaining bodily or mental control and well-being.